Community-Based Health Research

Issues and Methods

Dr. Daniel S. Blumenthal is principal investigator for the Prevention Research Center at Morehouse School of Medicine. He is professor and chair of the school's Department of Community Health and Preventive Medicine and associate dean for Community Programs. He is a graduate of Oberlin College and the University of Chicago School of Medicine. He completed his residency in pediatrics at Charity Hospital of New Orleans (Tulane Division) and received his master of public health degree from Emory University. He is board certified in both pediatrics and preventive medicine.

Dr. Ralph J. DiClemente is the Charles Howard Candler Professor of Public Health and associate director, Emory Center for AIDS Research. He holds concurrent appointments as professor in the School of Medicine, Department of Pediatrics, Division of Infectious Diseases, Epidemiology, and Immunology; and the Department of Medicine, Division of Infectious Diseases; and the Department of Psychiatry. He was most recently chair, Department of Behavioral Sciences and Health Education at the Rollins School of Public Health, Emory University. Dr. DiClemente was trained as a health psychologist at the University of California San Francisco where he received his PhD in 1984 after completing an MSPH in Behavioral Sciences at the Harvard School of Public Health and his undergraduate degree at the City University of New York. Dr. DiClemente has published extensively in the area of HIV/STD prevention, particularly among adolescents and young adults. He has authored more than 200 articles, chapters, and books.

Community-Based Health Research

Issues and Methods

Daniel S. Blumenthal, MD, MPH,
Ralph J. DiClemente, PhD

Editors

 Springer Publishing Company

Springer Publishing Company, Inc.
536 Broadway
New York, NY 10012-3955

Acquisitions Editor: Sheri W. Sussman
Production Editor: Jeanne W. Libby
Cover design by Joanne E. Honigman

03 04 05 06 07/5 4 3 2 1

Library of Congress Cataloging-in-Publication Data

Community-based health research : issues and methods / Daniel S. Blumenthal, Ralph J. DiClemente, editors.
   p. cm.
Includes bibliographical references and index.
ISBN 0-8261-2025-3
   1. Community health services—Research.   2. Health promotion.   3. Outcome assessment (Medical care)
RA425.C7375 2004
362.1'2'072—dc21   2004045732

Printed in the United States of America by Integrated Book Technology.

To Gina and my mom

Ralph DiClemente

To Marjorie and my dad

Daniel Blumenthal

Contents

Contributors

Nabih R. Asal, PhD
Professor and Director
Division of Epidemiology
Department of Health Policy and
  Epidemiology
College of Medicine
University of Florida
Gainesville, Florida 32608

Laura A. Beebe, PhD
Department of Biostatistics and
  Epidemiology
College of Public Health
University of Oklahoma Health
  Sciences Center
Oklahoma City, OK

Richard A. Crosby, PhD
Rollins School of Public Health
Department of Behavioral
  Sciences and Health
  Education and Emory Center
  for AIDS Research
Emory University
Atlanta, GA 30322

Andrea Cruz
Director, Southeast Georgia
  Communities Project
Lyons, GA 30436

Sharon K. Davis, MEd, MPA,
  PhD
Social Epidemiology Research
  Division
Department of Community
  Health and Preventive
  Medicine and the
  Cardiovascular Research
  Institute
Morehouse School of Medicine
Atlanta, GA 30310

Kirk W. Elifson, PhD
Department of Sociology
Georgia State University
University Plaza
Atlanta, GA 30303

Caswell Evans, DDS, MPH
National Institutes of Health
Bethesda, MD 20892

David Holtgrave, PhD
Rollins School of Public Health
Department of Behavioral
  Sciences and Health
  Education and Emory Center
  for AIDS Research
Emory University
Atlanta, GA 30322

Deborah Holtzman
Division of Adult and Community
   Health
Centers for Disease Control and
   Prevention
Atlanta, GA 30333

Bill Jenkins, PhD, MPH
Centers for Disease Control and
   Prevention
Atlanta, GA 30333

Camara Jones, MD, PhD
Centers for Disease Control and
   Prevention
Atlanta, GA 30333

D. N. Yung Krall
PO Box 33391
Decatur, GA 30033

Fred Murphy, MSPH
4112 Fieldway Road
Rex, GA 30273

Nana Nyarko
Lakewood Heights
   Redevelopment Corp.
Atlanta, GA 30315

Catlainn Sionean, PhD
Behavioral Interventions and
   Research Branch
Division of STD Prevention
Centers for Disease Control and
   Prevention
Atlanta, GA 30333

Claire E. Sterk, PhD
Chair, Department of Behavioral
   Sciences and Health
   Education
Rollins School of Public Health
Emory University
Atlanta, GA 30322

Elleen Yancey, PhD
Morehouse School of Medicine
Atlanta, GA 30310

FOREWORD

In issuing the 1997 apology to the survivors of the Tuskegee Syphilis Study, President Bill Clinton said, "we commit to increase our community involvement so that we may begin restoring lost trust." Honoring that commitment is the key to conducting community-based research ethically and effectively.

Conducting research in the community requires both the application of sound scientific methodology and the recognition of the role of the community in all aspects of the research. The latter includes participation in formulating the research question, examining the protocol, providing feedback on the results, and reviewing drafts of manuscripts. Collaborating with the community entails a variety of considerations, including an understanding of the Tuskegee Study and its meaning to the community, ethnic minority views of health professionals and research, and an anticipation of community responses to health promotion interventions.

More recent federal research programs have recognized the commitment to increase community involvement and have revised their requirements for conducting community-based research to ensure community participation. The Centers for Disease Control's REACH (Racial and Ethnic Approaches to Community Health) initiative has put research dollars in the hands of community organizations in projects exploring ways to reduce health disparities. The agency's Extramural Prevention Research Program has made meaningful community participation a requirement for funding. The 26 Prevention Research Centers funded by CDC "conduct participatory, community-based research to prevent disease and promote health," according to their statement of purpose. Each center is required to have an active Community Advisory Board.

CDC is not the only federal agency sponsoring community-based research. The budget of the National Institutes of Health doubled from $13.6 billion in 1998 to $27.3 billion in 2003, and it continues to increase.

Most of the NIH dollars support basic research, but in the last few years, increasing amounts have underwritten community-based research. This is entirely appropriate, because universities need to develop more balanced research portfolios. Important basic science discoveries continue to take place in our university laboratories but those discoveries have not benefitted large segments of our population.

For instance, although we are well aware of the damage done by cigarette smoke and the mechanisms of this damage, we are still struggling to discover effective ways to dissuade young people from starting to smoke. We know well the risks that are associated with obesity and sedentary lifestyles as well as the biochemistry and physiology of those risks, but we have not yet found successful strategies to promote better nutrition and more physical activity. AIDS and other sexually transmitted diseases continue to plague us, and although we know how they are transmitted and how they do their damage at the molecular level, we have not discovered how to prevent their transmission on a population-wide basis. These and many similar topics are the legitimate subjects of community-based research.

Community-based research is where medicine, public health, and science meet. Put another way, community-based research gives medicine the information it needs to serve communities as well as individuals and gives public health the science base that it has needed for so long in the field of health promotion. Medicine and public health, which have grown apart for too long, can reunite in part by joining in community-based research.

The editors of this book have attempted to bring together in one place a description both of epidemiologic methods and a discussion of community-level issues. It is a volume that will prove useful to those who wish to conduct contemporary community-based research.

David Satcher, MD, PhD
Former Surgeon General
Washington, D.C.

Part I

Issues

Chapter 1

COMMUNITY-BASED RESEARCH: AN INTRODUCTION

Daniel S. Blumenthal and Elleen Yancey

Community-based research is scientific inquiry involving human subjects that takes place in the community—that is, outside of the laboratory, hospital, or clinic setting. It is the "fourth estate" of research, assuming its station relatively recently alongside basic, clinical, and health services research. It guides public-health workers who are engaged in improving the health of populations just as traditional clinical research guides the actions of clinicians in caring for individual patients.

Beyond the aspect of location, community-based research is defined by several other concepts:

- *Prevention focus:* Community-based research may describe the epidemiology of a disease or condition, identify risk factors, or test a health promotion intervention, but (unlike laboratory or hospital- or clinic-based research) it does not generally evaluate new modes of therapy. Health problems can be identified and assessed on a community-wide basis; prevention-related messages or policies can be tested across a community; but in general, treatment of disease can only be delivered and evaluated on an individual basis.

- *Population-centered:* Community-based research focuses on a population rather than on individuals. The population that is the unit of interest may be a geographically defined community, a group with a common personal characteristic (i.e., age, race, sex, occupation), or a group with a common modifiable risk factor (i.e., tobacco use, risky sexual behavior). If the study involves a health promotion intervention, the intervention may be directed at one individual at a time, but the analysis is still done at the population level.

• *Partnership with the community:* The contemporary approach to community-based research does not countenance conducting research *on* a community, or even *in* a community, but rather *with* a community, in a partnership arrangement (Green, Daniel, & Novick, 2001). Depending on the approach to creating and sustaining the partnership, community-based research is sometimes called participatory research (Stoecker & Bonacich, 1992, 1993), action research (Brown & Tandon, 1984), participatory action research (Whyte, 1991), community research (Hatch et al., 1993), or other similar designations. This feature of community-based research has its basis in both ethical and pragmatic considerations and is the subject of additional discussion later in this chapter.

• *Multidisciplinary approach:* The methods of community-based research include those of the biomedical sciences, the behavioral sciences, and the social sciences, and approaches from more than one discipline are often combined in a single project. Typically the members of a research team will represent a number of disciplines. This sometimes leads scientists whose perspective encompasses a single discipline to view community-based research as lacking rigor, but well-conducted community-based research is as rigorous as any other type of well-conducted research.

• *Participants continue their usual activities:* Participants in community-based research must be reached where they live or work—in their natural surroundings. This means that they may be exposed to a variety of confounding influences. For instance, adolescents participating in a school-based trial of an intervention to prevent tobacco use may also see antismoking messages on television and billboards and may receive tobacco-related information in church, in after-school activities, or elsewhere. If smoking rates decline, it may be difficult to identify the cause or causes. This is unlike the situation of the laboratorian, whose subjects may live in a cage or a petri dish, and unlike that of the clinical trials specialist, who can be fairly certain that his or hers is the only experimental drug being administered to the subject.

• *Motivation to participate may be low:* Taking part in a prevention-oriented research project often represents a low priority for potential participants. Their incentive to participate is quite different from that of ill persons in a therapeutic trial or even an etiologic study. This is especially the case in a low-income community, where top priority is assigned to finding the means to pay the rent or put a meal on the table. Consequently, attrition rates may be high in community-based studies (Blumenthal, Sung, Williams, Liff, & Coates, 1995).

PUBLIC HEALTH AND COMMUNITY-BASED RESEARCH

Community-based research is differentiated from traditional clinical research in the same way that public health is differentiated from clinical medicine: in the former of each of these dyads, the focus is on a population; in the latter, it is on the individual. Community-based research advances the science of public health, just as clinical research advances the science of clinical medicine. Community-based research and public health are so closely linked that an understanding of the function and history of public health is needed in order to understand community-based research.

An oft-quoted definition of public health is that of C-E. A. Winslow, published in 1949:

> Public health is the science and art of preventing disease, prolonging life, and promoting physical and mental health through organized community efforts for the sanitation of the environment, the control of community infections, the education of the individual in the principles of personal hygiene, the organization of medical and nursing services for the early diagnosis and treatment of disease, and the development of the social machinery which will ensure to every individual in the community a standard of living adequate for the maintenance of health. (Winslow, 1949)

In short, public health is the sum of the activities undertaken collectively to promote the health of society. Improving the practice of public health is the mission of community-based research, and in many ways the history of public health is the history of community-based research.

HISTORY OF PUBLIC HEALTH AND COMMUNITY-BASED RESEARCH

Public Health Through the Nineteenth Century

Medicine has its origins in the mists of prehistory. It was advanced beyond shamanism by semimythical figures such as Hippocrates,

Aesculapius, and Imhotep. The profession of nursing has its roots in the Middle Ages, in Catholic orders that were developed to meet the needs of the Crusaders. However, public health—the population-based concept of health and illness—did not begin to develop until the seventeenth and eighteenth centuries.

The London merchant John Graunt might be considered the first public-health figure of note. On the suggestion of his friend William Perry, he collected the best mortality figures available as a volume entitled *Natural and Political Observations upon the Bills of Mortality* (1662) and thus developed an approach to evaluating the health of populations. He noted that the death rate among males was greater than among females, that mortality was higher in urban than in rural areas, and that death rates varied by season (Burton, Smith, & Nichols, 1980, p. 17).

Bernardino Ramazzini, the Father of Occupational Health, published *De Morbis Artificum Diatriba* (Discourse in the Diseases of Workers) in 1700. This document examined workers as a population and described the conditions to which they are prone.

In 1779, the Scotsman James Lind, a surgeon in the British Royal Navy, performed perhaps the first important community-based investigation. At that time, scurvy (now known to be a vitamin C deficiency disorder) was a major problem among sailors. Lind demonstrated the value of citrus fruit in scurvy by administering it to sailors who had the disease and comparing its effect with that of other alleged remedies (cider vinegar, elixir of vitriol, sea water, and spices), which were given to other groups of scorbutic sailors. Only the sailors given citrus recovered (Burton et al., 1980, p. 20). Lind's study was particularly remarkable because up to that time, little of what was known or believed in medicine had been derived from experimentation. Approaches to treating and preventing disease were based on anecdote and the experience of leading physicians. Although Lind approached the problem of scurvy from a therapeutic perspective, the Admiralty subsequently ordered the dispensing of citrus juice and fruit as a preventive measure, resulting in the disappearance of scurvy from the British Navy.

Edward Jenner demonstrated in 1798 that innoculation with the benign cowpox virus conferred immunity to smallpox, setting the stage for twentieth-century advances in immunization and the eradication of smallpox. Edwin Chadwick, in 1842, pointed out the effect of sanitation on the health of the public in his report, *The Sanitary Condition of the*

Labouring Population of Great Britain. This document led to the passage of the Public Health Act of 1848, the creation of a General Board of Health, the appointment of Medical Officers of Health, and the establishment of a number of legal provisions controlling sanitation, water supplies, and housing.

The obstetrician and anesthesiologist John Snow's legendary status as the "first epidemiologist" stems from his role in controlling the London cholera epidemic of 1854. By mapping cases of the disease and comparing the incidence rates among persons served by the city's two water companies, he became convinced that the disease was spread via water obtained by the public from the Broad Street pump. He recommended to the authorities that the handle be removed from the pump, and when this was done, the epidemic subsided (Centers for Disease Control [CDC], 2001).

Biology and medicine by this time were advancing through the application of research methods rather than by anecdote and speculation. Louis Pasteur (1822–1895) and Robert Koch (1843–1910) established the discipline of microbiology. Their methods were taken up by others, who identified the agents and modes of transmission of infectious diseases of all varieties. But this research was chiefly laboratory-based. Population-based prevention research was still to be developed.

Until the late nineteenth century, public health was primarily based on sanitary measures that could be implemented as a matter of policy, without participation on the part of the public. Improving the public's health by teaching the principles of hygiene and sanitation to those who stood to benefit became one of the mainstays of public health nursing as it evolved. In 1880, New York City established a Division of Child Hygiene in the New York Health Department. This division demonstrated that public health nurses could reduce infant mortality through home visiting and teaching (State of Missouri, 2001). Lillian Wald was the leading figure in the development of the profession of public health nursing (Nursingworld, 2001) and thus became one of the pioneers of public health education.

In 1869, Massachusetts established the first state board of health and other states soon followed. The first local health departments were established in 1911 in Yakima County, Washington, and Guilford County, North Carolina (Burton et al., 1980, pp. 32–33). State and local health departments became the mainstay of public health, collecting health-related statistics, controlling infectious disease, and providing health education to the public.

Federal Research Initiatives

In 1887, a one-room Laboratory of Hygiene was established at the Marine Hospital on Staten Island. This grew and became the National Hygienic Laboratory, later renamed the National Institute of Health, and relocated to Bethesda, Maryland. A 1912 act of Congress authorized it to

> study and investigate the diseases of man and conditions influencing the origin and spread thereof including sanitation and sewage, and the pollution directly or indirectly of navigable streams and lakes of the United States and may from time to time issue information in the form of publications for the use of the public. (Hanlon & Pickett, 1984)

Thus was created what was to become the world's largest and greatest health and disease research establishment, authorized to conduct research in the community as well as in the laboratory and the clinic. The agency was subdivided into specialized institutes, each focused on a disease or set of diseases, and its name was pluralized in 1948 to become the National Institutes of Health (NIH). Now comprised of 27 separate institutes and centers and an annual budget of over $18 billion, it conducts research on its own clinical campus and funds research at universities and other research establishments through a program of grants and contracts. Little of this research, however, is community-based; almost all of it is either basic bench research or clinical studies performed in the hospital or ambulatory setting.

A national public health agency, the Centers for Disease Control and Prevention (CDC), was established in Atlanta, Georgia, in 1946 as the Communicable Disease Center. Originally created to control malaria in the southeastern United States, its mission was later broadened to include communicable disease generally. As the focus of public health enlarged to include noncommunicable disease, CDC broadened its mission as well, expanding to include 12 centers, institutes, and offices devoted not only to communicable disease control but also to the prevention of chronic disease, injury, occupational disorders, environmental problems, and birth defects.

Historically, the work of CDC has been in the area of public health practice, conducting disease surveillance and providing assistance to state and local health departments. It is only in recent years that the agency has explicitly begun to fund and conduct research. Its extramural research efforts include a $15 million Prevention Research Initiative (fiscal year 1999) (PHPPO, 2001) and Prevention Research Centers Program funded at about $30 million. Through these initiatives, federal grants specifically for community-based prevention research have become available. In addition, CDC conducts a substantial volume of intramural community-based research.

Public Health in the Twentieth and Twenty-First Centuries

Through the mid-twentieth century the major task of public health was to contain infectious disease through measures aimed at sanitation, hygiene, and immunization. By the middle of the century, however, morbidity and mortality patterns in the U.S. and other developed countries had changed. Infectious diseases were no longer the leading causes of death; this distinction now belonged to heart disease, cancer, stroke, pulmonary disease, and trauma (Table 1.1). Unlike infectious disease, the etiology of these conditions is multifactorial. They cannot be prevented with a simple immunization or, in most cases, be cured with a drug. Primary prevention of these conditions depends in large part on behavior change: changes in diet, exercise, tobacco and alcohol use, and employment of safety measures such as automobile seat belts. Their secondary prevention depends on access to, and participation in, screening programs for conditions such as hypertension and breast, cervical, and colorectal cancer.

Public health then began to turn its attention to these conditions by offering programs of public health education and screening. Little was known, however, about the efficacy of various health-education modalities or about the best ways to cover a population with screening services. Health messages could be transmitted via the mass media, presented on posters, taught in school—but which of these, if any, were effective in promoting behavior change? Screening programs could be mounted in public health clinics—but how could they be made to reach the people who needed them and how could treatment be assured to those whose screening tests were positive? Questions such as these became the focus of community-based research.

Epidemiologists and other prevention scientists began to undertake large community-based investigations. One of the first observational studies was the notorious Tuskegee Syphilis Study (1932–1972) in which 399 African American men in rural Alabama were denied treatment for syphilis in order to document the natural history of the disease

TABLE 1.1   Leading Causes of Death, 1900 and 1997

1900[a] Rank and cause of death	% of all deaths	1997[b] Rank and cause of death	% of all deaths
1. Pneumonia and influenza	11.8	1. Heart disease	31.4
2. Tuberculosis (all forms)	11.3	2. Cancer	23.3
3. Diarrhea and enteritis	8.3	3. Stroke	6.9
4. Diseases of the heart	8.0	4. Chronic obstructive pulmonary disease	4.7
5. Intracranial vascular lesions	6.2	5. Unintentional injuries	4.1
6. Nephritis	4.7	6. Pneumonia and influenza	3.7
7. Unintentional injuries	4.2	7. Diabetes mellitus	2.7
8. Malignant neoplasms	3.7	8. Suicide	1.3
9. Certain diseases of early infancy	3.6	9. Kidney disease	1.1
10. Diphtheria	2.3	10. Liver disease	1.1

[a]Wallace and Everett, 1986
[b]CDC, 1997a

(Jones, 1993). The consequences of this misguided effort are discussed in chapter 3.

The Framingham Study (Kannel, 2000) was (and is) a prospective observational study of cardiovascular disease that enrolled most of the population of the town of Framingham, Massachusetts, in 1948 and has followed them, their children, and new arrivals ever since. An enormous amount of information on the epidemiology and risk factors (a term coined by the study) of coronary disease, stroke, peripheral artery disease, and heart failure was generated; a 2001 MEDLINE search for published papers on the Framingham Study since 1966 identified more than 500 references in English and multiple other languages.

The Framingham study was followed by community intervention trials (chapter 10) that attempted to alter the incidence and prevalence of cardiovascular disease and its risk factors through health promotion interventions. One of the first was the oft-cited cardiovascular disease prevention project in the North Karelia Province of Finland (Puska et al., 1985). In the United States, the Stanford Three-City Project (Farquhar et al., 1977) was followed by the Five-City Project (Farquhar et al., 1985). Other notable community intervention trials directed at risk factors for cardiovascular disease included the Minnesota Heart Health Program (Mittelmark et al., 1986), COMMIT (Community Intervention Trial for Smoking Cessation) (COMMIT Research Group, 1995a, 1995b), and the Pawtucket Heart Health Program (Carleton, Lasater, Assaf, Feldman, & McKinley, 1995).

Toward the end of the twentieth century, attention was brought to bear on longstanding racial and ethnic disparities in health status in the U.S. Mortality rates for nearly every major cause of death are greater for African Americans than for Whites, and other racial minorities suffer disproportionately high mortality from certain diseases and conditions (Table 1.2). These disparities are related to poverty, but they are not wholly the result of poverty. To a major extent, they represent a "prevention gap." In most cases, prevention is more effective than medical care in improving health. All of the leading causes of death are largely preventable, but minorities are less likely than Whites to receive needed preventive services. Largely unknown are the interventions and programs most likely to succeed in preventing disease and promoting

TABLE 1.2 Mortality Rates for Selected Diseases by Ethnic Group, 1995
Deaths Per 100,000 Population

	White	Black	Hispanic	Native American
All causes	476.9	765.7	386.8	468.5
Heart Disease	133.1	198.8	92.1	104.5
Cancer	127.0	171.6	79.7	80.8
Stroke	24.7	45.0	20.3	21.6
Unintentional Injury	29.9	37.4	29.8	56.7
Homicide	5.5	33.4	15.0	11.9
Diabetes	11.7	28.5	19.3	27.3
HIV Infection	11.1	51.8	23.9	7.0

Note: From CDC, 1997b

health among minority populations (Blumenthal & Yancey, 2000). Community-based prevention research to explore these issues is still in its early stages.

The case of breast cancer is instructive. Screening for breast cancer with mammography is known to reduce mortality. Breast cancer incidence is higher among white women than among black women, but breast cancer mortality and stage at diagnosis are higher in blacks than whites, and five-year survival rates are lower in blacks. These patterns suggest that a program of mammography in African-American women would reduce or eliminate the black-white disparities, yet the CDC Behavioral Risk Factor Surveillance System showed that in 1997, only 76.1% of black women over the age of 50 had obtained a mammogram in the preceding two-year interval (Boelen, Rhodes, Powell-Griner, Bland, & Holzman, 2000).

COMMUNITY-BASED RESEARCH AND COMMUNITY INVOLVEMENT

New Paradigms

Traditionally, the relationship between health professional and patient/client has reflected a substantial power differential; a patient has been expected to follow "doctor's orders." This has been equally true whether the health professional was a clinician or a public health worker and regardless of whether the interaction was around practice or research.

Now, both medical care and public health are undergoing a transformation. Many patients expect that their physicians will include them as partners in the therapeutic relationship, sharing information on the risks and benefits of treatment options so that physician and patient can develop a management plan together (Blumenthal, 1996). In traditional clinical research, individual participants (the term "subjects" is losing favor) must be fully informed of the potential risks and benefits of the research and must give their consent in writing to participate. At each institution receiving federal research funds, an Institutional Review Board (IRB) must review every proposed research project to insure that it meets all ethical standards. Although a set of federal regulations (45CFR46) laying out these requirements has existed since the mid-1970s, it is only in recent years that it has been well-enforced.

In the field of public health, the patient or client is the community, and a similar shift in the professional-client paradigm is underway.

Public health workers are now less likely to view the community as a population that must be immunized and sanitized, and much more likely to recognize it as a partner and a participant in promoting its own health. This is especially true in community-based research, where both ethics and research rigor demand that the community serve as a partner. Of course, federally-funded community-based research is subject to the same ethical requirements as other research involving humans and must be approved by the appropriate IRB.

Community-based research often takes place in minority and other disadvantaged communities, and this is likely to become an even more frequent venue in the future as research scientists address racial and ethnic health status disparities. These are often powerless communities that are accustomed to being the purported beneficiaries of health and social programs over which they have no control. Organized to participate with public health workers and researchers as partners in finding better ways to improve their health, they can become empowered to take action on other issues, such as education, transportation, or housing. In the broad sense, these are also public health issues.

Levels of Community Participation

Typically, community leaders are convened as an "advisory board" to offer input to researchers on a research agenda or on a particular project. Depending on the researchers' approach, this can be a meaningful or a sham relationship. Hatch and colleagues identify four levels or models of community participation (Hatch et al., 1993). At the first level, the persons consulted by the researchers are at the periphery of the community, often working for human service agencies and living outside the community. In this model, community residents are unaware of the purpose of the research and have no influence on its design.

At the second level, the project's advisors are leaders drawn from organizations and churches within the community, but the researchers retain total control of the project. In this model, there is community involvement, but it is passive.

At the third level, community leaders are asked not only for endorsement of the project, but for guidance in hiring community residents to serve as interviewers, outreach workers, etc. This model is "community based but not community involved, since community members do not contribute to the design of the research nor do they have a significant role in interpreting findings." This model may also offer potential for manipulation of the community, since those hired are often influential members of the local cultural systems.

The fourth level both involves and empowers the community. In it, community representatives are first among equals in defining the research agenda, identifying the problem to be studied, analyzing its contributory factors, and proposing possible solutions. The community "negotiates, as a collaborator, the goals of the study, the conduct of the study, and the analysis and use of study findings."

At this fourth level, there are likely to be conflicts and differences between the researchers and the community. The challenge to the researchers is to negotiate these differences and build a trusting relationship with the community rather than to search for another, more compliant, venue in which to implement their plans. This relationship between community and researcher is the most difficult to attain but one that is most conducive to conducting effective and ethical community-based research.

COMMUNITY ORGANIZING
FOR PARTNERSHIP DEVELOPMENT

Several models offer guidance for partnering with the community as part of a community health planning (not necessarily research) process. These include, for instance, the World Health Organization's "Healthy Communities" Program (Hancock, 1993) and CDC's "Planned Approach to Community Health" (PATCH) (Goodman, Steckler, Hoover, & Schwartz, 1993). Braithwaite and colleagues (Braithwaite, Murphy, Lythcott, & Blumenthal, 1989) describe a model of "community organization and development for health promotion" that borrows from the "empowerment education" approach of Paulo Friere (1968). They list seven steps in the model as guidance to health educators or community organizers:

1. *Learning the community layout:* Entry to the community should be preceded by a study of community geography, health status measures, etc.
2. *Learning the community ecology:* This includes identifying places where people congregate as well as meeting community leaders and "gatekeepers" and learning their relationship to each other.

3. *Community entry process:* The process must be negotiated with gatekeepers, and the community organizer must be "validated" by the formal and informal community networks.
4. *Building credibility:* Tangible resources, such as jerseys for a neighborhood football team, are helpful at this step.
5. *Development of a community coalition board:* The board described in this step is one that is consumer-dominated (at least 60%) but also includes academic, agency, and organizational representatives as well as elected officials.
6. *Conducting a community needs assessment:* This involves a survey or similar methods to identify those health issues felt by community residents to be most important. In the context of a research initiative, this step might be entitled *"Establishing a research agenda."*
7. *Planning the intervention:* Again, in the context of a research initiative, this would be *"Planning the research project."* Implicit is the need to provide feedback on the results of the project or the intervention to the community.

Principles for Working With Communities

Among those that have published principles for sustaining working relationships between academic institutions and communities is the organization, *Community-Campus Partnerships for Health* (1997):

1. Partners must agree on missions, goals, and outcomes
2. Partners should have mutual trust, respect, and commitment.
3. Partnerships need to build on identified strengths and assets. Instead of approaching a community-based partnership solely by itemizing all of the problems that the community faces, the partners should also identify their strengths and assets.
4. Good partnerships should have clear communication among partners and transparency in the decision-making process.
5. Partnerships evolve using feedback to, among, and from all partners.
6. Roles, norms, and processes for the partnerships should evolve from the input and agreement of all partners. Partnerships need a governance structure that establishes a common understanding of how to proceed.

7. Successful partnerships have relationships with local leaders and funding agencies.
8. Effective partnerships use existing structures, such as schools and worksites, to incorporate solutions into their mission.

Principles of Community-Based Research

Israel, Schultz, Parker, and Becker (1998) identify eight principles of community-based research that are based on the assumption that the researchers will build an appropriate relationship with the community:

1. *Recognizes community as a unit of identity.* This acknowledges that a community may be a geographic entity but alternatively may be defined by some other commonality among members, such as ethnicity or occupation.
2. *Builds on strengths and resources within the community.* As in the Principles for Partnerships, above, this recognizes that public health workers and researchers have often described communities by their needs and problems, but a more contemporary approach to community health needs assessment calls for an inventory of the community's assets as well (Sharpe, Greaney, Lee, & Royce, 2000). "Assets" may include businesses, churches, schools, organizations, agencies, and so forth.
3. *Facilitates collaborative partnerships in all phases of the research.* Communities should share control over all phases of the research process: problem definition, data collection, interpretation of results, and application of the results.
4. *Integrates knowledge and action for mutual benefit of all partners.* Results of community-based research should not be simply added to the broad base of knowledge of community health, but should also be integrated into local efforts at community change.
5. *Promotes a co-learning and empowering process that attends to social inequalities.* Researchers and community members learn from each other. Moreover, researchers recognize the inherent inequality between themselves and community members and attempt to address this factor by sharing information, decision-making power, resources, and support.
6. *Involves a cyclical and iterative process.* This cycle proceeds from partnership development and maintenance through community assessment, problem definition, development of research methodol-

ogy, data collection, analysis, and interpretation, through dissemination of results, determination of action and policy implications, taking action, and establishing mechanisms for sustainability. By implication, the process would then start over.

7. *Addresses health from both positive and ecological perspectives.* The former is the more limited model of health that emphasizes physical, mental, and social well-being. The latter recognizes the role of economic, cultural, historical, and political factors.

8. *Disseminates findings and knowledge gained to all partners.* This emphasizes sharing the results of the research with community partners in understandable language and includes the need to consult with participants prior to submission of manuscripts for publication, acknowledging the contributions of participants, and developing co-authored publications when appropriate.

CULTURAL COMPETENCE IN COMMUNITY-BASED RESEARCH

Partnering or creating a coalition with a community presupposes that the researcher is competent to communicate and interact with persons who are part of the community's culture; that is, the researcher should be culturally competent. Cultural competence begins with understanding the concepts of culture, values, beliefs and ethnicity, from both the individual and organizational systems perspectives. It is important to understand the impact and influence of cultural competence on one's own cultural perspective as it relates to community-based research. *Culture* is an arrangement of behavior patterns that enables a society to reach collective achievement. These patterns of behaviors are transmitted by symbols such as cars, houses, clothing and academic degrees and are specific to particular groups of people. Culture shapes how people experience their world and make decisions on quality of life and work (Health Resources and Services Administration, 1998).

Values are abstract concepts of worth. They are not initially an individual's own concepts, but are social products of what has been taught or imposed upon the person and slowly, over time, internalized. As an individual matures and/or is exposed to other values, he may consciously adopt the value or may discard or modify it to fit his own perspectives.

Beliefs are structures of values, common language and similar life experiences shared within a culture. *Ethnicity* refers to groups of people generally believed to be biologically related and who share a unique social and cultural heritage.

Most definitions of *cultural competence* describe an increased cultural awareness and knowledge and a change in attitude. The concept is multifaceted; researchers and practitioners must view it broadly in order to assimilate it and put it into practice. Cross, Bazon, Dennis, and Isaacs (1989) have developed the following definition of cultural competence that contains the essential principles:

> A set of attitudes, skills, behaviors, and policies that enable organizations and staff to work effectively in cross-cultural situations. It reflects the ability to acquire and use knowledge of the health-related beliefs, attitudes, practices, and communication patterns of clients and their families to improve services, strengthen programs, increase community participation, and close the gaps in health status among diverse population groups. Cultural competence also focuses attention on population-specific issues including health-related beliefs and cultural values (the socioeconomic perspective), disease prevalence (the epidemiological perspective), and treatment efficacy (the outcome perspective).

A culturally competent system acknowledges and incorporates, at all levels, the importance of culture, the assessment of cross-cultural interactions, vigilance toward the dynamics that result from cultural differences, expansion of cultural knowledge and adaptation of services, and research and prevention models to meet culturally unique needs. Cultural competence is a developmental process and should be viewed as a goal that institutions, agencies and individuals strive to achieve.

Cross (1988) constructed a cultural competency continuum that identifies stages of development (Figure 1.1).

The first point, *Cultural Destructiveness* is the most negative end of the continuum. It is represented by attitudes, policies and practices that are destructive to cultures and individuals within them. These are

Cultural Destructiveness → Cultural Incapacity → Cultural Blindness → Cultural Precompetence → Basic Cultural Competence → Advanced Cultural Competence

FIGURE 1.1 Cultural competency continuum.

extreme programs and individuals that actively participate in purposeful destruction of a culture, assuming that one race is superior and should eradicate "inferior cultures" because of their perceived lower position. These entities are actively involved in services that deny people access to their natural helpers or healers. They remove children from their families based on race and purposely risk the well being of minority individuals in social or medical experiments without their knowledge or consent.

Cultural Incapacity, the second point on the continuum, does not incorporate intentional cultural destructiveness, but rather a lack of capacity to work effectively with diverse groups. There is extreme bias and the belief in racial superiority of the dominant group. Frequently there is a disproportionate application of resources, support of racist policies, maintenance of stereotypes and lower expectation of minorities.

At the third point, *Cultural Blindness,* research is conducted and health services provided with the intent of being unbiased. The belief prevails that culture makes no difference, e.g., "all people are the same." Research and health services approaches traditionally used by the dominant culture are universally applied. Cultural blindness ignores the cultural strengths of individuals and groups and encourages assimilation into the majority culture. Minorities are viewed from the cultural deprivation model that asserts problems are the result of inadequate resources rather than cultural differences.

Cultural Pre-Competence, point four, implies movement toward competence. Weaknesses are recognized and attempts to improve practices and increase knowledge are made. There is a danger of "tokenism," however, as systems attempt to explore more culturally competent processes. Precompetent entities often lack information on what is possible and how to proceed. These systems and individuals are characterized by the desire to practice culturally competent services and a commitment to the rights of individuals.

Point five, *Basic Cultural Competence,* is characterized by acceptance of and respect for difference, continuing self-assessment regarding culture, and careful attention to the dynamics of difference. There is a continuous expansion of cultural knowledge and resources and a variety of adaptations to research and health services, adjusting and creating new models in order to address more effectively the needs of multiple populations.

Advanced Cultural Competence, point six, is the most positive end of the continuum. It is characterized by holding culture in high esteem and seeking to add to the knowledge base of cultural competence by conducting culture-based research, examining intra-cultural phenomena as opposed to comparison research, which compares minority populations to the dominant population.

There are three primary arenas of change where development can and must occur if there is to be a movement toward cultural competence: (1) Attitudes change to become less ethnocentric and biased; (2) Policies change to become more flexible and culturally impartial; and (3) Practices change to become more congruent with the culture(s) with which the interaction is based.

Culturally Competent Research

Culturally competent research should encompass the following components: awareness and acceptance of cultural differences; awareness of one's own cultural values; understanding of the dynamics of difference; basic knowledge about the culture of the population involved in the research; knowledge of the research participants' environment; ability to adapt research methods, evaluation, and data collection; and analysis to fit the participants' cultural context.

The Culturally Competent Researcher

In addition to the characteristics of culturally competent research, there are five elements the characterize the culturally competent *researcher.*

1.   Acknowledges cultural differences and becomes aware of how they affect the research process. While all people share common basic needs, there are vast differences in how people of various cultures go about meeting these needs. It is necessary to understand and accept that each culture finds some behaviors, interactions and values more important or desirable than others. The researcher should develop a dual perspective, i.e., an understanding of his/her own culture and appreciation of differences among others.

2.   Recognizes the influence of one's own culture on perspectives. Acknowledges how cultural norms and values have shaped day-to-day behaviors and have been reinforced by families, peers and social institutions.

3.   Understands and accepts the dynamics of difference. When researchers of one culture interact with and collect data from partici-

pants of another culture both groups bring their own unique history and the influence of current political and socioeconomic power relationships to the research interaction.

4.   Makes a conscious effort to understand the meaning of the data within his/her own cultural context as well as that of the participants. It is important to understand the results from both perspectives. Qualitative research methods often effectively enhance the interpretation of quantitative data. Interview and focus groups can be utilized to effectively clarify survey results, providing indepth perspectives to unanswered questions. It is important to understand what symbols are meaningful and what they mean to research participants, how health is defined and how peer group and family group networks are configured.

5.   Knows where and how to obtain detailed information regarding the culture of populations involved in the research. Gains enough knowledge to know how to seek information, what information to seek, and how to apply it effectively.

Culturally competent research strengthens the effectiveness of researchers, health care providers, and health service systems by providing them with accurate information to improve their work. It also empowers diverse communities by equipping them with the knowledge and skills to understand health care issues and to intervene on their own behalf (National Center for Cultural Competence, 2000).

SUMMARY

Community-based research is the force that propels modern public health. Advances against the most important causes of morbidity and mortality in industrial societies and, hence, major gains in life expectancy, will depend on scientific advances at the community level. Moreover, improvements in public health at the community level offer the best chance of reducing or eliminating racial and ethnic health status disparities.

Community-based research relies on the same scientific principles as other types of research. The processes by which hypotheses are developed and tested and considerations of study design are essentially in any type of research. There are, however, an important set of considerations that apply uniquely to community-based research.

These include the principles that govern relationships between researchers and communities and the principles of cultural competence that prepare researchers to create the community partnerships needed to conduct community-based research.

REFERENCES

Blumenthal, D. S., Sung, J., Williams, J., Liff, J., & Coates, R. (1995). Recruitment and Retention of Subjects for a Longitudinal Cancer Prevention Study in an Inner-city Black Community. *Health Services Research, 30,* 197–205.

Blumenthal, D. (1996). Quality of care: What is it? *New England Journal of Medicine, 335,* 891–894.

Blumenthal, D. S., & Yancey, E. M. (2000). Poverty, race, and prevention. *Journal of Medical Association of Georgia, 89,* 42–45.

Boelen, J. C., Rhodes, L., Powell-Griner, E. E., Bland, S. D., & Holtzman, D. (2000, March 24). State-specific prevalence of selected health behaviors, by race and ethnicity—Behavioral risk factor surveillance system, 1997. *Morbidity and Mortality Weekly Report, 49*(SS02), 1–60.

Braithwaite, R. L., Murphy, F., Lythcott, N., & Blumenthal, D. S. (1989). Community Organization and Development for Health Promotion within an Urban Black Community: A Conceptual Model. *Health Education, 20*(5), 56–60.

Brown, L. D., & Tandon, R. (1983). Ideology and political economy in inquiry: Action research and participatory research. *Journal of Applied Behavioral Science, 19,* 277–294.

Burton, L. E., Smith, H. H., & Nichols, A. W. (1980). *Public health and community medicine* (3rd ed.). Baltimore: Williams and Wilkins.

Carleton, R. A., Lasater, T. M., Assaf, A. R., Feldman, H. A., & McKinlay, S. (1995). The Pawtucket Heart Health Program: Community changes in cardiovascular risk factors and projected disease risk. *American Journal of Public Health, 85*(6), 777–785.

COMMIT Research Group. (1995a). Community Intervention Trial for Smoking Cessation (COMMIT): I. Cohort results from a four-year community intervention. *American Journal of Public Health, 85*(1), 183–193.

COMMIT Research Group. (1995b). Community Intervention Trial for Smoking Cessation (COMMIT):II. Changes in adult cigarette smoking prevalence. *American Journal of Public Health, 85*(1), 193–200.

CDC, National Center for Health Statistics. (1997a). National Vital Statistics System and unpublished data.

CDC, National Center for Health Statistics. (1997b). Health United States 1996–97 and Injury Chartbook. Hyattsville, MD.

CDC: http://www.cdc.gov/ncidod/dbmd/snowinfo.htm. Accessed September 23, 2001.

Community-Campus Partnerships for Health. (1997). *Principles of good partnerships.* San Francisco. Access at: http://futurehealth.ucsf.edu/ccph/principles.html#principles

Cross, T. L. (1988). Services to minority populations: Cultural competence continuum. *Focal Point, 3*(1), 1–2.

Cross, T., Bazon, B., Dennis, K., & Isaacs, M. (1989). *Towards a culturally competent system of care, (I)*. Washington, DC: Georgetown University Child Development Center CASSP Technical Assistance Center.

Farquhar, J. W., Fortmann, S. P., Maccoby, N., Haskell, W. L., Williams, P. T., Flora, J. A., et al. (1985). The Stanford Five-City Project: design and methods. *American Journal of Epidemiology, 122*(2), 323–334.

Farquhar, J. W., Maccoby, N., Wood, P. D., Alexander, J. K., Breitrose, H., Brown, B. W. Jr., et al. (1977). Community education for cardiovascular health. *Lancet, 1*(8023), 1192–1195.

Freire, P. (1970). *Pedagogy of the oppressed.* New York: Herder and Herder.

Goodman, R. M., Steckler, A., Hoover, S., & Schwartz, R. (1993). A critique of contemporary community health promotion approaches: based on a qualitative review of six programs in Maine. *American Journal of Health Promotion, 7*(3), 208–220.

Green, L., Daniel, M., & Novick, L. (2001). Partnerships and Coalitions for Community-Based Research. *Public Health Reports,* Supplement 1, 116, 20–31.

Hancock, T. (1993) The evolution, impact and significance of the healthy cities/ healthy communities movement. *Journal of Public Health Policy, 14*(1), 5–18.

Hanlon, J. J., & Pickett, G. E. (1984). *Public health administration and practice* (8th ed., pp. 37–38). St. Louis: Times Mirror/Mosby.

Hatch, J., Moss, N., Saran, A., Presley-Cantrell, L., & Mallory, C. (1993). Community research: Partnership in black communities. *American Journal of Preventive Medicine, 9*(6 Suppl), 27–31.

Health Resources and Services Administration, Bureau of Primary Health Care, U.S. Department of Health and Human Services. (1998). *Cultural Competence: A Journey.* Washington, DC: Author.

Israel, B. A., Schulz, A. J., Parker, E. A., & Becker, A. B. (1998). Review of community-based research: Assessing partnership approaches to improve public health. *Annual Review of Public Health, 19,* 173–202.

Jones, J. H. (1993). *Bad blood.* New York: Free Press.

Kannel, W. B. (2000). The Framingham Study. ITS 50-year legacy and future promise. *Journal of Atherosclerosis & Thrombosis, 6*(2), 60–66.

Mittelmark, M. B., Luepker, R. V., Jacobs, D. R., Bracht, N. F., Carlaw, R. W., Crow, R. S., et al. (1986). Community-wide prevention of cardiovascular disease: Education strategies of the Minnesota Heart Health Program. *Preventive Medicine, 15,* 1–17.

National Center for Cultural Competence. (2000, Summer). *Cultural competence in primary health care: Partnerships for a research agenda* (Policy Brief No. 3). Washington, DC: Goode, T. & Harrisone, S.

Nursingworld.org: http://www.nursingworld.org/hof/waldld.htm Accessed September 23, 2001.

PHPPO: http://www.phppo.cdc.gov/eprp/default.asp. Accessed September 23, 2001.

Puska, P., Nissinen, A., Tuomilehto, J., Salonen, J. T., Koskela, K., McAlister, A., Kottke, T. E., Maccoby, N., & Farquhar, J. S. (1985). The community-based strategy to prevent coronary heart disease: Conclusions from the ten years of the North Karelia Project. *Annual Review of Public Health, 6*(1), 147–193.

Sharpe, P. A., Greaney, M. L., Lee, P. R., & Royce, S. W. (2000, March–June). Assets-oriented community assessment. *Public Health Reports, 115*(2–3), 205–211.

State of Missouri: http://www.health.state.mo.us/Publications/100-20.html Accessed September 23, 2001.

Stoecker, R., & Bonacich, E. (Eds.). (1992). Participatory research, Part I. *American Sociology, 23*, 3–115.

Stoecker, R., & Bonacich, E. (Eds.). (1993). Participatory research, Part II. *American Sociology, 24*, 3–126.

Wallace, R. B., & Everett, G. D. (1986). The prevention of chronic illness. In J. M. Last (Ed.), *Maxcy-Rosenau Public Health and Preventive Medicine* (12th ed., p. 1126). Norwalk, CT: Appleton-Century-Crofts.

Whyte, W. F. (1991). *Participatory action research.* Newbury Park, CA: Sage.

Winslow, C.-E. A. (1949). The evolution of public health and its objectives. In J. S. Simmons (Ed.), *Public health in the world today.* Cambridge, MA: Harvard University Press.

Chapter 2

Assessing and Applying Community-Based Research

Caswell Evans

As public-health leaders and decision makers, we need to have confidence in our practices, programs, and services. Yet, all too often there are little or no data sufficient to evaluate the effectiveness of our community-based interventions. There are high expectations concerning public health services, their proper application and value. The public wants to feel safeguarded from health risks and have assurance that tax dollars are focused on priority needs. The community and elected leaders hold public health officials accountable for appropriate expenditure of funds. At the same time, we want to know whether the services we provide and the programs we conduct are effective. We wonder whether an alternative approach might achieve improved outcomes. Despite these concerns, there is a paucity of reliable information that enables informed decisions to be made concerning competing options for program design, or comparing one program approach to another. There is too little information to guide decisions about program content, structure, or application based upon documented evidence of the effectiveness of those options or programs, when assessed by valid scientific methods and reported in the scientific literature.

COMMUNITY PREVENTIVE SERVICES TASK FORCE

The work of the U.S. Community Preventive Services Task Force is changing that picture. The task force has developed recommendations for community-level interventions intended to prevent disease, disability, and injury, and to protect health, based upon the strength of evidence found in the pertinent literature. The essential questions are not complex: What is the evidence that a public health program is effective in achieving its intended disease prevention objectives? Under what conditions and circumstances have program approaches proven effective? Does evidence point to ineffective practices that consequently cannot be recommended? Furthermore, if data indicate that a program is effective, what can be said about the cost of the intervention? Does the level of effectiveness appear to justify the expenditure of resources relative to what was achieved (Pappaioanou & Evans, 1994)?

The application of evidence-based assessments of the effectiveness of population-focused programs and services is still in its formative stages; however, evidence-based decision making has been developing in other areas of health care (McGinnis & Foege, 2000). From a public health perspective, the potential for utilization of recommendations emanating from such assessments is substantial. In the United States, public health programs and services are conducted by more than 50 states and territories, and by more than 3,000 city or county local jurisdictions. In addition, organized health systems, such as health maintenance organizations (HMOs), have great interest in population-based measures to ensure improved health for their enrolled population and surrounding communities.

The interest in, and use of, evidence-based recommendations to guide decisions in the health care of *individuals* was advanced considerably by *The Guide to Clinical Preventive Services* issued by the U.S. Preventive Services Task Force (USPSTF) in 1989 with subsequent revisions (USPSTF, 1996). That guide serves to inform health care practitioners about the demonstrated effectiveness of clinical interventions intended to prevent disease in individual patients. The USPSTF conducted extensive reviews of the literature covering more than 100 clinical interventions intended to prevent 70 illnesses and conditions. Based upon review of the evidence, recommendations were made regarding the provision of primary and secondary clinical preventive measures, such as screening, immunization, chemoprophylaxis, and counseling, for patients in clinical settings.

However, since the work of the USPSTF focused on preventive measures applied to patients in a clinical setting, population-based and applied measures were not considered, such as those intended to prevent disease among large groups of people in community, occupational, or school settings. Subsequently, public health leaders and others concerned about population health recognized the value of a similar approach that could result in better informed guidance for selecting, funding, and implementing community-based preventive services.

In 1992, in order to test the feasibility of this approach, the Centers for Disease Control and Prevention (CDC) conducted a pilot project to study methods to assess the evidence of the effectiveness of public health interventions. During 1994 and 1995, the Council on Linkages between Academia and Public Health Practice—supported by a health philanthropy and in collaboration with federal, state, and local public health leaders—conducted a more extensive assessment of the feasibility of this approach and also tested methods for evaluating scientific evidence upon which guidelines for community-based disease prevention interventions could be founded. The council concluded that "the potential benefits of public health practice guidelines are immediate and far reaching" (Council on Linkages between Academia and Public Health Practice, 1995; Novick, 1997). Taking action on these findings, the CDC convened the *Task Force on Community Preventive Services.* This task force was charged with taking the earlier findings and recommendations to the next level and developing evidence-based guidance for preventive interventions intended for application among populations. The product of this effort would be the *Guide to Community Preventive Services.*

Representation on the task force was necessarily broad in order to assure the diversity of knowledge and experience needed to succeed in the effort. The task force included representation from numerous disciplines (such as maternal and child health, infectious and chronic disease control, environmental health, and substance abuse prevention), and several levels of public health practice and interest (such as state and local public health departments, behavioral and social sciences, epidemiology, primary care, health systems management, and health policy).

GUIDE TO COMMUNITY PREVENTIVE SERVICES

The Guide to Community Preventive Services is intended to provide a base of information and support for decisions concerning population-based interventions to prevent disease and promote and protect health. Such guidance is helpful for several reasons. Health decision-makers value evidence that is based on science to substantiate their practice and choice of procedure or intervention. However, the scientific literature is vast, varies in its consistency and quality, and requires time and analysis that is beyond the reach of most practitioners. Moreover, the informed conclusions of experts who have taken the time to labor through the scientific evidence in a systematic manner is rarely available to help inform a decision in a time frame that is pertinent to the issue or problem at hand (Truman et al., 2000). Consequently, the products of such evidence-based reviews provide useful information to inform decisions on health programs, intervention strategies, and policies regarding what has been shown to have been effective, and cost-effective, among a variety of operational settings and conditions.

The topics addressed in the guide were initially taken from the Healthy People 2000 initiative (U.S. Department of Health and Human Services [DHHS], 1991), and later on the Healthy People 2010 initiative (DHHS, 2000), and from the paper by McGinnis and Foege (1990) on the actual causes of death in the United States. Topics were also selected for their breadth of impact upon the population overall; the burden of the disease, injury, impairment, or exposure; preventability and the range of potential interventions; risk behaviors with large collective effects on health; those conditions with the largest effects upon health across the lifespan; and the usefulness of the selected topics for the target audience. (Truman et al., 2000; Zaza, Wright-Aguero, et al., 2000). Consequently, each chapter would include a description of the significance of the health problem in terms of the population's burden of disease; would justify the selection of the intervention evaluated; would present the evidence of the effectiveness of the interventions, based upon a rigorous systematic review of the scientific literature; would make recommendations based upon the evidence; and would explain the link between the evidence and the recommendation. Each chapter would also identify important research gaps identified in the literature to inform future research efforts and stimulate interest in specific subjects for research.

Of course, any practitioner, program director, policy maker, or other person using the findings and recommendations of the guide would still need to assess the information in light of their own community and local circumstance, and assess the level of fit between information in the guide and the parameters of the specific situation in question.

Subjects addressed in the guide were organized within three sections: changing risk behaviors; reducing diseases, injuries, and impairments; and addressing environmental and ecosystem challenges.

Changing risk behaviors addresses activities that also affect other health-related outcomes. Topics addressed in this section include

- Tobacco use
- Alcohol abuse and misuse
- Other addictive drugs
- Physical activity
- Nutrition
- Sexual behavior

Topics that relate to reducing the effects of specific diseases, injuries, and impairments are addressed in a second section under the following subject headings:

- Cancer
- Diabetes
- Vaccine-preventable diseases
- Improved pregnancy outcomes
- Oral health
- Motor vehicle occupant injury
- Injuries due to violence
- Mental impairment and disability/mental health services

To ensure that the importance of the physical, biological, and socio-cultural environments were considered, the third section is focused on sociocultural environment.

Each chapter includes practical examples of how evidence-based findings on the effectiveness of interventions intended to improve or protect the health of populations could prove useful. Recent problems involving immunizations among school children in some urban centers illustrate situations where evidence of successful approaches else-where could inform and improve program planning. The guide's chapter on vaccine-preventable diseases is intended to be an instructive and useful tool in such matters (Task Force on Community Preventive Services, 2000; Briss, Rodewald, et al., 2000).

USING VACCINATIONS AS AN EXAMPLE OF THE PROBLEM

The following vignette provides an example of the potential applicability of the vaccine-preventable disease chapter. Although in the United

States there is general acceptance of the value of vaccinations and most people are seen periodically in health care settings, unfortunately vaccination opportunities are missed. In addition, parents and caretakers give numerous reasons for not taking children for their immunizations. Among them are perceptions that the child is healthy and does not need immunizations; that vaccine-preventable childhood diseases are rare and when they do occur are not serious; that time cannot be taken from work, immunizations are not affordable, and the parents were never advised that their children needed immunizations. For some, there are religious objections as well. Although information regarding the damaging effects of childhood diseases and the protective value of vaccinations is available and often promoted to inform parents about the importance of immunizations, low levels of immunization still persist in some communities.

In December 2000, the District of Columbia Public Schools learned that 40,000 of the system's 68,500 students were out of compliance with vaccination standards. The urgency of the situation was apparent and parents of unimmunized children were given a year to get their children properly vaccinated.

At the end of 2001, the District school system found that 19,000 school children still lacked complete immunizations despite the year-long campaign (Operation Final Push, 2002). The school board then proclaimed that any child not fully immunized by the end of January 2002 would be excluded from school. Multiple entities responded by launching initiatives to address the problem. With no evidence base to guide them, however, they could only offer programs that intuitively seemed appropriate.

Media covered the problem and numerous community organizations worked to inform parents about the immunization requirements. More than two dozen immunization sites, including mobile clinics, were opened, with extended hours of service. In collaboration with local radio stations, a contest was proposed to encourage competition among schools, with the school producing the largest percentage of fully immunized children to be declared the winner. Rewards of free movie tickets were considered for children who completed their immunizations and submitted the appropriate documentation.

The recent closure of D.C. General Hospital added to the logistical challenges of providing the necessary immunizations. However, the D.C. Healthcare Alliance, a coalition of health care facilities, agencies, and insurers formed after the closure of D.C. General Hospital, rallied resources in order to deliver immunizations to those who are poor and uninsured. Staffing difficulties and overtime expenses of operating the expanded clinics were additional burdens for the involved organizations (Operation Final Push, 2002). Immunization clinics sponsored by the D.C. Department of Health were overflowing their capacity.

The record-keeping system of the school district contributed to the problem. It was estimated that as many as half the children without proof of immunization had actually been fully immunized; however, their immunization records had been misfiled or lost within the school system and the family had no documentation. The school district had a centralized database into which practitioners could enter immunization records, but relatively few practitioners knew about and utilized the centralized data system (Blum, 2002).

By the end of January 2002, 4,500 school children still were not fully immunized, and these children were turned away from school and prohibited from returning until they had complete documentation of their immunizations (Blum & Wilgoren, 2002). A month later the problem had been reduced to only a few hundred children.

Other cities and public health jurisdictions have faced similar problems. Washington, D.C. is not alone. This is only one example of how the best intentions of public health efforts may not produce the desired outcomes. However, for many public health interventions there is an available body of evidence that demonstrates the effectiveness of planned interventions. The outcome of an assessment of this evidence could be used as a resource for developing programs or services based upon interventions that were proven effective in other locations. The challenge is to structure the assessment of the evidence and data in such a way that a high level of confidence can be placed upon the findings, and consequently upon the recommendations derived from them. From such an assessment we can become better informed about what interventions have proven effective, in what settings, for what populations, and under what conditions, so that we can choose more wisely among interventions with demonstrated effectiveness. Were such information available, interventions could be planned with a higher degree of confidence in their overall effectiveness. It is this challenge that the Community Preventive Services Task Force undertook.

STRUCTURE AND PROCESS

The structure and process of the task force's approach to assessing the evidence of the effectiveness of community-based disease prevention interventions has been presented in the literature (Briss, Rodewald, et al., 2000; Truman et al., 2000; Zaza, Lawrence, et al., 2000; Zaza, Wright-Aguero, et al., 2000), and task force recommendations regarding other interventions have also been published (Task Force on Community Preventive Services, 2000, 2001a, 20001b, 2002a, 2002b, 2002c). The following provides a brief review of the approach taken by the task force. The reader is encouraged to review the cited reference works for a more detailed presentation of this information.

To facilitate communication and assure common frames of reference, the task force agreed on several important definitions. These definitions provided consistency of meaning for the task force and could be useful for application in other settings as well. The definitions (Truman et al., 2002) follow:

- Community: A group of individuals who share one or more characteristics.
- Community Preventive Service: An intervention that prevents disease or injury or promotes health in a group of persons.
- Determinant: A causal factor that is hypothesized to affect health outcomes, for example, demographic and population factors; environmental factors; social, economic, educational, health care, cultural, or other systems; or preventive interventions.
- Effectiveness: Improvement in health or behavioral outcomes produced by an intervention in a community setting.
- Evidence-based method: A strategy for linking public health recommendations to the underlying scientific evidence that demonstrates effectiveness.
- Health outcomes: Measure of health or loss of health that includes
    - mortality—rates of death, years of potential life lost; quality adjusted life years gained, disability adjusted life years lost;
    - morbidity—disease or injury rates, infertility rates, disability, chronic pain, functional status, psychiatric disorders;
    - pregnancy and birth rates.

- Intermediate outcome: Biological markers and behavioral variables that occur in the pathway between a determinant and the final health outcome. For example, levels of risk behaviors; rates of access to, usage of, and extent of preventive services; physiologic measures (blood pressure or cholesterol); and levels of environmental exposures. To put this into perspective, it is important to note that one health outcome (diabetes) can lead to another health outcome (cardiovascular disease), making the earlier health outcome an "intermediate" outcome.

• Public health practitioners: Persons responsible for providing public health services, regardless of the organizational setting in which they work. This definition includes a wide variety of health workers in public health agencies, managed care or community health center settings, and academic institutions, among others. (U.S. Public Health Service, 1997)

METHODS

The process of developing the evidence-based *Guide to Community Preventive Services* entailed a series of specific and rigorous steps. The methodology was stringent to ensure a uniform approach to the various chapter subjects, with consistent application of logic and decision making. A chapter development team was identified for each chapter. Depending on the subject, 4 to 10 individuals who were experts in the field were asked to participate in developing each chapter. This ensured breadth of knowledge of the subject matter, the usefulness and relevance of the conceptual approach to the chapter, and reduced the likelihood that important information or issues would be overlooked, while also reducing opportunities for the chapter to be influenced by errors of interpretation of identified information (Briss, Zaza, et al., 2000).

Next, logic frameworks, as shown in Figure 2.1, were structured to diagram the chain of hypothesized causal relations among determinants, intermediate outcomes, and final outcomes. The logic frameworks also provided the chapter development teams with a structure that enabled them to identify which public health intervention would be useful to achieve a public health objective and where in the framework it might exert its effect. Once interventions were identified, a detailed analysis was developed for each intervention to identify the hypothetical links between the intervention and the health outcomes. These analyses provided a more in-depth assessment of the various linkages that comprised a logic framework. The analytic frameworks also furnished initial guidance for evaluating the linkages and directing the team's initial search for evidence.

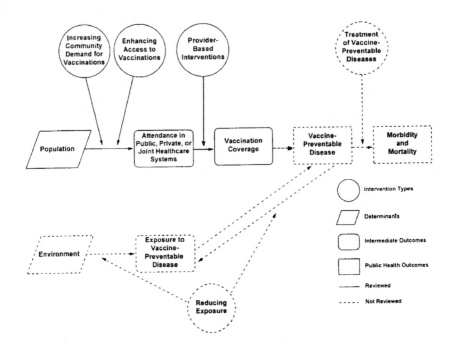

FIGURE 2.1   Example of a logic framework.

The selection of types of interventions to assess in chapters was influenced by the following considerations (Briss, Rodewald, et al., 2000):

- potential for reducing the burden of disease or injury
- potential for increasing healthy behaviors and reducing unhealthy behaviors
- potential to increase the utilization of effective interventions that are not widely applied
- potential to decrease or eliminate less effective interventions in favor of more effective, or cost-effective, interventions
- current level of interest among providers, experts in the field, and decision makers

A systematic search and retrieval of the pertinent literature was the next step. The detailed analyses served to identify the essential inclusion criteria used in searching for evidence by identifying particular interventions and specifying particular outcomes. Other criteria included years in which studies were conducted (older studies were not included) and restricted the search to English-language publications. Evidence had to demonstrate that an intervention would improve health outcomes at the population level. The effect could be direct (for example, community water fluoridation is shown to reduce the occurrence of dental caries in a community) or indirect (for example, increasing tobacco sales taxes to increase tobacco prices could reduce tobacco use, which could reduce related mortality and morbidity) (Briss, Rodewald, et al., 2000).

As evidence of the effectiveness of interventions was identified, detailed information pertaining to the evidence was categorized and entered onto a standardized abstract form (Zaza, Lawrence, et al., 2000). In this way, evidence that met the inclusion criteria was assessed to identify clearly the intervention studied, the context in which the intervention was applied, the study design, quality of the study, and the results. Two separate reviewers validated the categorization of this information and any discrepancies were brought to the attention of the chapter development team for resolution. In this process, the suitability of each study design for assessing the effectiveness of interventions was assessed using agreed-upon standards. In this way, studies were classified as having greatest, moderate, or least suitable study designs for assessing effectiveness (see chapter 5 for a review of study designs).

For example, studies using concurrent comparison groups and a prospective measurement of exposure and outcome were classified as having the greatest suitability of study design (Briss, Rodewald, et al., 2000) (Table 2.1).

All retrospective study designs or multiple pre- or postmeasurement designs without comparison groups were classified as having moderate suitability. Single pre- and postmeasurement study designs without concurrent comparison groups or exposure and outcome measures in a single group at the same point in time were classified as least suitable.

Quality of execution of the study was also assessed by considering various threats to validity, including study population and intervention descriptions, sampling, exposure and outcome measurement, data analysis, and interpretation of results (Briss, Rodewald, et al., 2000). Categories of specific procedural limitations and weaknesses were identified pertinent to the various threats to validity (Zaza, Lawrence,

TABLE 2.1 Suitability of Study Design for Assessing Effectiveness in the *Guide to Community Preventive Services*

Suitability	Attributes
Greatest	Concurrent comparison groups and prospective measurement of exposure and outcome
Moderate	All retrospective designs or multiple pre- or postmeasurements but no concurrent comparison group
Least	Single pre- and postmeasurements and no concurrent comparison group or exposure and outcome measured in a single group at the same point in time

Note: From Briss, Zaza, et al., 2000.

et al., 2000), and studies were classified as having good, fair, or limited quality of execution based upon the number of documented limitations. For example, studies were classified as having good execution if they had 0–1 limitations in their execution. Studies with 2–4 limitations were classified as fair, and those with 5 or more were classified as limited. Results across a group of related studies were assessed and described qualitatively and statistically using median and range or interquartile range of effect sizes. The body of evidence of effectiveness was then classified as strong, sufficient, or insufficient based on the number of studies available, the strength of their design and execution, and the size and consistency of the reported effects (Briss, Rodewald, et al., 2000).

In the rare circumstance where evidence was not available and the intervention was considered important enough, or was practiced widely and a recommendation had to be made, the task force agreed to use expert opinion. However, this option was never utilized. The summary of factors utilized to assess the strength of a body of evidence pertaining to population-based interventions is shown in Table 2.2 (Briss, Rodewald, et al., 2000).

In the final presentation of findings, interventions that demonstrated stronger evidence of effectiveness received stronger recommendations. The relationship between the findings regarding strength of evidence and the strength of recommendation is shown in Table 2.3 (Briss, Rodewald, et al., 2000).

Evidence that was found to be inconsistent in effect size or direction—based upon definable characteristics of the study population,

TABLE 2.2 Assessing the Strength of a Body of Evidence on Effectiveness of Population-Based Interventions in the *Guide to Community Preventive Services*

Evidence of effectiveness[a]	Execution— good or fair[b]	Design Suitability— greatest, moderate, or least	Number of studies	Consistent[c]	Effect size[d]	Expert opinion[e]
Strong	Good	Greatest	At least 2	Yes	Sufficient	Not used
	Good	Greatest or moderate	At least 5	Yes	Sufficient	Not used
	Good or fair	Greatest	At least 5	Yes	Sufficient	Not used
		Greatest			Large	Not used
			Meet Design, Execution, Number, and Consistency Criteria for Sufficient but Not Strong Evidence			
Sufficient	Good	Greatest	1	Not applicable	Sufficient	Not used
	Good or fair	Greatest or moderate	At least 3	Yes	Sufficient	Not used
	Good or fair	Greatest or moderate or least	At least 5	Yes	Sufficient	Not used
Expert Opinion	Varies	Varies	Varies	Varies	Sufficient	Supports a recommendation
Insufficient[f]	A. Insufficient designs or execution		B. Too few studies	C. Inconsistent	D. Small	E. Not used

[a]The categories are not mutually exclusive; a body of evidence meeting criteria for more than one of these should be categorized in the highest possible category.
[b]Studies with limited execution are not used to assess effectiveness.
[c]Generally consistent in direction and size.
[d]Sufficient and large effect sizes are defined on a case-by-case basis and are based on task force opinion.
[e]Expert opinion will not be routinely used in the *Guide* but can affect the classification of a body of evidence as shown.
[f]Reasons for determination that evidence is insufficient will be described as follows: A. Insufficient designs or executions, B. Too few studies, C. Inconsistent. D. Effect size too small, E. Expert opinion not used. These categories are not mutually exclusive and one or more of these will occur when a body of evidence fails to meet the criteria for strong or sufficient evidence.
Note: From Briss, Zaza, et al., 2000.

TABLE 2.3   Relationship of Strength of Evidence of Effectiveness and Strength of Recommendations

Strength of Evidence of Effectiveness	Recommendation
Strong	Strongly recommended
Sufficient	Recommended
Insufficient empirical information supplemented by expert opinion	Recommended based on expert opinion
Insufficient	Available studies do not provide sufficient evidence to assess
Sufficient or strong evidence of ineffectiveness or harm	Discouraged

Note: From Briss, Zaza, et al., 2000.

setting, or the intervention—led to separate recommendations for different settings. For example, an intervention might be recommended for application in a health department but not in a managed care setting. Contradictory or insufficient evidence of effectiveness of an intervention in any setting or population would lead to a determination of insufficient evidence to assess effectiveness. Evidence of ineffectiveness, absent any evidence of effectiveness in a definable setting, led to a recommendation against application of the intervention. Evidence of unintended outcomes of interventions, both positive and negative outcomes, was also assessed (Briss, Rodewald, et al., 2000).

With this information, chapter development teams considered the findings and recommendations in terms of their applicability by

- defining target populations and settings most suitable for the intervention;
- determining whether the available studies evaluated the intervention in those settings;
- assessing the extent to which study settings might be representative of the larger target population;
- making judgments about whether the intervention worked better in one population or setting than in others. (Briss, Rodewald, et al., 2000)

Where possible, economic analysis of interventions was also conducted in order to assess the resource implications of interventions and facilitate decision making concerning resource allocation to achieve maximal health improvement (Garande-Kulis et al., 2000).

Based upon this information, the task force then determined how widely the resulting recommendations should apply and made recommendations regarding further research needed in the subject area.

EXAMPLES OF INTERVENTION RECOMMENDATIONS: VACCINATIONS

Let's return to the discussion and example of the problem of vaccinations among school-aged children in Washington, D.C. Although the problem might not have been totally avoided, it could have been ameliorated possibly by application of interventions shown to have been effective in similar settings and directed at a similar population. This is where the findings and recommendations of the Community Preventive Services Task Force could be applied with the understanding that each of the recommended interventions has documented effectiveness in similar settings and populations. It is important to remember that the effectiveness of vaccines is not at issue; the challenge at issue is to identify and apply community-based interventions that result in more at-risk persons receiving needed vaccines. (The recommendations of the task force concerning vaccinations are directed towards improving coverage in children, adolescents, and adults, and are not limited to school children. Even so, the recommended interventions have general applicability to schoolchildren and several are particularly relevant to this age group.)

Task force recommendations on immunization programs are organized under three subject headings: increasing community demand; enhancing access to vaccine services; and provider-based interventions.

Increasing Community Demand for Vaccinations

• Client reminder/recall: This intervention entails reminding members of a target population that vaccinations are due (reminders) or late (recall). Such interventions are *strongly recommended* based on the strength of the scientific evidence of their effectiveness in improving vaccine coverage among children and adults, in a range of settings and populations, when applied at the individual level as well as the community level, and whether used alone or as part of a multicomponent intervention. (Task Force on Community Preventive Services, 2000)

• Multicomponent interventions that include education: These are interventions that provide knowledge to the target population, and perhaps providers of vaccines, and use at least one other action to improve vaccine coverage. Such interventions are *strongly recommended* based on strong evidence that they improve coverage among children and adults, improve coverage in a broad range of applications that include community-wide and clinic settings, and have incorporated education and other actions. It should be pointed out that the relative contribution of specific elements of multicomponent interventions could not be clearly determined. (Task Force on Community Preventive Services, 2000)

• Vaccine requirements for child care, school, and college attendance: Such requirements are in the form of laws or policies that require vaccination or proof of immunity as a condition of attendance. These types of requirements were *recommended* based on sufficient evidence that such requirements are effective in reducing vaccine-preventable diseases or improving vaccine coverage, and that such requirements are effective in all relevant target populations. However, the relative differences in degrees of effectiveness among various laws and policies, or their enforcement, in different jurisdictions could not be determined. (Task Force on Community Preventive Services, 2000)

• Community-wide education-only interventions: These interventions only provide education to target populations and providers in a geographic area. The task force found *insufficient evidence* to assess the effectiveness of such interventions due to few studies with limited designs that showed inconsistent results. (Task Force on Community Preventive Services, 2000)

• Clinic-based education-only interventions: Such interventions only provide education directed towards populations served by a public health or medical clinic. The task force found *insufficient evidence* to assess the effectiveness of such interventions due to few studies with limited designs that showed inconsistent results. (Task Force on Community Preventive Services, 2000)

• Client or family incentives: Incentives could be a financial or other motivator or could be in the form of penalties that stimulate persons to obtain vaccinations. The task force found too few studies, focused on various incentives, and demonstrating variability in the size of the results. Consequently, it found that *insufficient evidence* existed to assess the effectiveness of client or family incentives to improve vaccine coverage. (Task Force on Community Preventive Services, 2000)

• Client-held medical records. These interventions are records that are retained by members of a target population or their families that indicate which vaccinations have been received. Again, the task force found *insufficient evidence* to assess the effectiveness of such interventions due to few studies with limited designs that showed inconsistent results. (Task Force on Community Preventive Services, 2000)

Enhancing Access to Vaccination

• Reducing out-of-pocket costs: In order to reduce the personal expense of vaccines, the costs could be paid by other sources, insurance coverage could be applied, and copayments for vaccinations could be reduced or eliminated. Such interventions are *strongly recommended* based on the strength of evidence that they improve vaccine coverage for children and adults, are effective in a range of settings and populations, are effective when applied at the individual and the population level, and whether used alone or as part of a multicomponent strategy. (Task Force on Community Preventive Services, 2000)

• Expanding access in health care settings: These are strategies that increase the availability of vaccines in public-health or medical clinic settings by reducing geographic barriers, expanding or changing hours of service, expanding the clinic settings in which vaccines are provided (for example, emergency rooms and subspecialty clinics), and developing new administrative procedures to provide vaccines such as express lines and drop-in clinics. Expanding access in health care settings is *strongly recommended* if the expansion is part of a multicomponent initiative, based on the strength of evidence that the result is improved vaccine coverage for children and adults in a range of health care settings. However, there was *insufficient evidence* to recommend expanded access only, due to the small number of studies with limitations in design and execution, reporting results with low effect sizes and statistically not significant. (Task Force on Community Preventive Services, 2000)

• Vaccination programs in women, infants, and children settings: These are efforts intended to improve vaccination among low-income participants of the supplemental nutrition program for eligible pregnant and postpartum women, their infants and children (the WIC program) where the service is provided in a nonmedical setting. Such interventions are *recommended* based on evidence that they are effective in improving vaccine coverage in children whether used alone or as part of a multicomponent initiative. (Task Force on Community Preventive Services, 2000)

• Home visits: These are interventions that entail a home visit and direct interaction with the child and family. Home visits can also involve telephone or mail reminders. Such interventions are *recommended* based on the evidence. However, these types of interventions are costly when compared to other forms of intervention intended to improve vaccine coverage. (Task Force on Community Preventive Services, 2000)

• Vaccine programs in schools: Such programs are intended to improve vaccine coverage of school-aged children by providing vaccine-related education and providing vaccinations or referrals in the school setting. Due to few studies assessing the effectiveness of school-based vaccine programs, the task force found *insufficient evidence* to make a recommendation regarding this form of intervention. (Task Force on Community Preventive Services, 2000)

• Vaccination programs in child care centers: These are programs focused on children of approximately 5 years and younger in child care settings. Due to the absence of studies, the task force found *insufficient evidence* to make a recommendation regarding this form of intervention. (Task Force on Community Preventive Services, 2000)

Provider-Based Interventions

• Provider reminder/recall: These are reminders for those who administer vaccines that they are due (reminder) or overdue (recall) for a specific patient or client. Reminders can be furnished via medical charts, computer flags, or other means. Provider reminders are *strongly recommended* based on the strength of evidence that they result in improved vaccine coverage for children, adolescents, and adults, whether used separately or in combination or as an element of a multicomponent intervention, and are effective in a range of settings and populations. (Task Force on Community Preventive Services, 2000)

- Assessment and feedback for vaccination providers: Such interventions entail retrospective evaluation and feedback concerning the performance of providers in delivering vaccinations to a client population. Based on the strength of evidence this form of intervention is *strongly recommended* and has been shown to be effective for children and adults. (Task Force on Community Preventive Services, 2000)
- Standing orders: This intervention involves non-physicians providing vaccines to a client population by protocol without direct physician involvement at the time of the service. Standing orders are strongly *recommended* based on the strength of evidence. (Task Force on Community Preventive Services, 2000)
- Provider education only: These are education efforts directed towards providers to increase their knowledge about vaccinations. Written materials, videos, lectures, and other forms of information delivery could be involved. Due to the small number of studies with limited design and execution, showing variable results, the task force found that *insufficient evidence* was available to assess the effectiveness of provider education alone as a means of increasing vaccine coverage for an at-risk population. (Task Force on Community Preventive Services, 2000)

DISCUSSION

As the vignette concerning the vaccine crisis in Washington, D.C. illustrated, there could be substantial benefit to developing population-based disease prevention, health promotion, and health protection interventions based on evidence of the effectiveness of interventions in other settings. The description of the methods used by the Community Preventive Services Task Force to assess, rate, and categorize the strength of evidence, leading to the development of evidence-based recommendations, provides a basis for understanding the complexity of such an undertaking. The detailed description of the vaccine-related recommendations from the task force provides an example of how evidence-based recommendations can be presented and focused on specific settings and community circumstances. Similar processes have led to task force recommendations concerning reduction of injuries to motor vehicle occupants pertaining to increasing child and adult safety-belt use and reducing alcohol-impaired driving (Task Force on

Community Preventive Services, 2001); reduction of tobacco use and exposure to environmental tobacco smoke (Task Force on Community Preventive Services, 2001); health care system and self-management education interventions to reduce morbidity and mortality from diabetes (Task Force on Community Preventive Services, 2002); increasing physical activity in communities (Task Force on Community Preventive Services, 2002); and prevention of dental caries, oral and pharyngeal cancers, and sports-related craniofacial injuries (Task Force on Community Preventive Services, 2002). As the task force completes its work regarding the full range of subjects under the headings of changing risk behaviors, reducing diseases, injuries, and impairments, and addressing environmental and ecosystem challenges, the magnitude of this undertaking can be readily discerned. It has boundless value to public health efforts to prevent disease and promote and protect health.

The recommendations, decisions, and actions of public-health leaders, policy makers, program planners, health program advocates, and many others can be informed by, and benefit from, the findings of community-based research. For example, because public-health strategies to increase vaccine levels among population groups is a constant challenge, such efforts can be strengthened by program planning that is based on evidence of what strategies have worked previously, among what populations, in what settings, and under what conditions. However, final decisions and actions about program concepts, content, and implementation must also be based on a firm understanding of local conditions, needs, resources, and priorities. Consequently, program decisions cannot be guided solely by research findings. Yet, evidence-based conclusions can lend powerful assistance when planning program features and in making choices among program options. The strength of the evidence can assist others in understanding the reasonable range of program outcomes so that expectations are neither too high nor too low. The evidence also provides an initial benchmark against which program performance can be assessed.

The process by which evidence-based findings were developed by the Community Preventive Services Task Force also illuminates the research process by identifying those aspects of research design and execution that lead toward reliable findings in the context of community-based research. In this way, research methods are informed and can be improved in the future. In addition, important gaps in knowledge can also be identified with the expectation that future research will be drawn to these gaps. This work provides an example of how systematic analysis of community-based research can benefit the health of the public. Interventions built upon the evidence of their effectiveness can improve attainment of public-health goals and objectives. Ultimately we can achieve greater success in preventing disease, promoting health, and protecting health in the community.

REFERENCES

Blum, J. (2002, January 25). DC Verifying immunizations. *The Washington Post,* p. B01.

Blum, J., & Wilgoren, D. (2002, January 29). 4,500 D.C. students locked out. *The Washington Post,* p. B01.

Briss, P. A., Rodewald, L. E., Hinman, A. R., Shefer, A. M., Strikas, R. A., Bernier, R. R., et al., and the Task Force on Community Preventive Services. (2000). Reviews of evidence regarding interventions to improve vaccination coverage in children, adolescents, and adults. *American Journal of Preventive Medicine, 18*(1S), 97–140.

Briss, P. A., Zaza, S., Pappaioanou, M., Fielding, J., Wright-De Aguero, L., Truman, B. I., et al., & the Task Force on Community Preventive Services. (2000). Developing an evidence-based guide to community preventive services—Methods. *American Journal of Preventive Medicine, 18*(1S), 35–43.

Council on Linkages between Academia and Public Health Practice. (1995, October). *Practice guidelines for public health: Assessment of scientific evidence, feasibility and benefits: A Report of the guideline development project for public health practice.* Washington, D.C.

Garande-Kulis, V. G., Maciosek, M. V., Briss, P. A., Teutsch, S. M., Zaza, S., Truman, B. I., et al., & the Task Force on Community Preventive Services. (2000). Methods for systematic reviews of economic evaluations for the guide to community preventive services. *American Journal of Preventive Medicine, 18*(1S), 75–91.

McGinnis, J. M., & Foege, W. H. (1990). Actual causes of death in the United States. *Journal of the American Medical Association, 270,* 2207–2212.

McGinnis, J. M., & Foege, W. (2000). Guide to community preventive services: Harnessing the science. *American Journal of Preventive Medicine, 18*(1S), 1–2.

Novick, L. F. (1997). Public health practice guidelines: A case study. *Journal of Public Health Management Practice, 3*(1), 59–64.

Pappaioanou, M., & Evans, C. A. (1994). Development of the guide to community preventive services: A U.S. Public Health Service Initiative. *Journal of Public Health Management Practice, 4*(2), 48–54.

Redfearn, S. (2002, January 15). Operation Final Push. *The Washington Post,* p. HE01.

Task Force on Community Preventive Services. (2000). Recommendations regarding interventions to improve vaccination coverage in children, adolescents, and adults. *American Journal of Preventive Medicine, 18*(1S), 92–96.

Task Force on Community Preventive Services. (2001a). Recommendations regarding interventions to reduce tobacco use and exposure to environmental tobacco smoke. *American Journal of Preventive Medicine, 21*(2S), 10–15.

Task Force on Community Preventive Services. (2001b). Recommendations to reduce injuries to motor vehicle occupants: Increasing child safety seat use, increasing safety belt use, and reducing alcohol-impaired driving. *American Journal of Preventive Medicine, 21*(4S), 16–22.

Task Force on Community Preventive Services. (2002a). Recommendations for healthcare system and self-management education interventions to reduce morbidity and mortality from diabetes. *American Journal of Preventive Medicine, 22*(4S), 10–14.

Task Force on Community Preventive Services. (2002b). Recommendations on selected interventions to prevent dental caries, oral and pharyngea cancers, and sports-related craniofacial injuries. *American Journal of Preventive Medicine, 23*(1S), 16–20.

Task Force on Community Preventive Services. (2002c). Recommendations to increase physical activity in communities. *American Journal of Preventive Medicine, 22*(4S), 76–72.

Truman, B. I., Smith-Akin, C. K., Hinman, A. R., Gebbie, K. M., Brownson, R., Novick, L. F., Lawrence, R. S., et al., and the Task Force on Community Preventive Services. (2000). Developing the guide to community preventive services—Overview and Rationale. *American Journal of Preventive Medicine, 18*(1S), 18–26.

U.S. Department of Health and Human Services. (1991). *Healthy people 2000: National health promotion and disease prevention objectives.* Washington, DC: DHHS, Public Health Service.

U.S. Department of Health and Human Services. (2000). *Healthy people 2010: Understanding and improving health and objectives for improving health* (2 vols). Washington, DC: U.S. Government Printing Office.

U.S. Preventive Services Task Force. (1996). *Guide to clinical preventive services* (2nd ed.). Baltimore: Williams & Wilkins.

U.S. Public Health Service. (1997). Public health workforce: An agenda for the 21st century. Washington, DC: U.S. Department of Health and Human Services.

Zaza, S., Lawrence, R. S., Mahan, C. S., Fullilove, M., Fleming, D., Isham, G. J., et al., & the Task Force on Community Preventive Services. Scope and organization of the guide to community preventive services. (2000). *American Journal of Preventive Medicine, 18*(1S), 27–34.

Zaza, S., Wright-De Aguero, L., Briss, P. A., Truman, B. I., Hopkins, D. P., Hennessy, M. H., et al., & the Task Force on Community Preventive Service. (2000). Data collection instrument and procedure for systematic reviews in the guide to community preventive services. *American Journal of Preventive Medicine, 18*(1S), 44–74.

Chapter 3

Public Health Ethics and Community-Based Research: Lessons from the Tuskegee Syphilis Study

Bill Jenkins, Camara Jones,
and Daniel S. Blumenthal

In 1895, one of the most important speeches in African-American history was delivered in Atlanta at the Cotton States Exposition. It proposed the development of African American communities by investments in self-help programs centered in Tuskegee, Alabama. This effort was called the Tuskegee Experiment. The speech laid the groundwork for support of self-development efforts in African American communities throughout the nation. Unfortunately, it also accepted segregation as a political reality. The speech became known as the Atlanta Compromise and established Booker T. Washington as the most influential African American leader of his day. In it he said, "Negroes and Whites may live as the hand, together in all things economic and separate in all things social." It was a trade-off that continues to plague Black leaders and their communities to this day.

Whether it was ethical to make this trade-off is also at the heart of the most tragic episode of medical and research misconduct in American history. This chapter is a review of that tragedy, which was entitled the Tuskegee Study of Untreated Syphilis in the Negro Male, more commonly called simply the Tuskegee Syphilis Study. Like Washington's speech, it continues to have an impact long after its conclusion. (The term "Tuskegee Experiment" is used in various writings to describe the Tuskegee development initiative of the early twentieth century, the training program for Black aviators conducted in Tuskegee during World War II, and the Tuskegee Syphilis Study. In this chapter, the term is reserved for the development initiative, and the notorious research project is called the Tuskegee Syphilis Study.)

BACKGROUND

With support of the leading philanthropists of the day, Booker T. Washington realized his dream of self-development for his people. Tuskegee Institute, later known as the Tuskegee Machine, produced a series of phenomenally successful programs and made Tuskegee the Camelot of Black America. It produced an agricultural program under George Washington Carver that saved the declining agricultural system of the South. It developed an architectural program in which students not only designed buildings and built them, but also made the bricks used in their construction.

The Tuskegee Machine also organized many segments of the Black community into powerful alliances, including the National Business and Professional League, the National Bar Association, the National Nurses Association, and the National Medical Association. It spawned the Negro Health Movement, which organized Negro Health Week in April of each year; this continues today as Public Health Week, focusing the nation on the health issues of the day. It also built and managed the only Black-owned and -managed hospital in the South (John Andrews Hospital, now closed) and trained the Tuskegee Airmen, who were World War II heroes. The real tragedy of this history is that today many people, including African Americans, ignore the significant achievements that were part of the Tuskegee Experiment and remember the one terrible tragedy. How is it that African Americans accomplished so many great things at Tuskegee and yet most people remember only the one bad thing associated with it?

Among those who heard Washington's speech was Julius Rosenwald, founder of the Sears department stores. One of the wealthiest men of his day, Rosenwald was fascinated by the development efforts that had gotten underway in Tuskegee only 30 years after the end of the Civil War. Through his foundation, Rosenwald became the chief underwriter of the Tuskegee Experiment—an experiment to see if African Americans could build a successful modern society in a small town in Alabama. The Rosenwald Fund provided monies not only to support Tuskegee Institute, but also to develop schools, factories, businesses, and agriculture.

By the end of World War I, the Tuskegee Experiment was in full swing under the leadership of Dr. Robert Moton, a Virginian who had succeeded Booker T. Washington as president of Tuskegee Institute. The son of former slaves, Moton was a graduate of Hampton Institute, where he had subsequently served for 25 years as the school's commandant in charge of military discipline (Moton, 1921).

The wartime draft had given the U.S. a new perspective on the health of its youth: shockingly high percentages of young male draftees, especially those from poor rural families, had failed their preinduction physical exams. Now, ironically, the health of American youth was being further damaged by the aftermath of the war. Many young men returning home were infected with syphilis, an often incurable and sometimes deadly infectious disease associated with social disruptions such as war.

By 1926, prevalence rates had reached 36% among the African American population of Macon County, where Tuskegee is located. Because of its relatively extensive resources and support from the Rosenwald Fund, Tuskegee was one of the few Black communities that could mount a syphilis treatment program. Such a program required substantial medical and logistical support because the treatment of syphilis necessitated an 8-week course of therapy with drugs containing toxic chemicals such as mercury and arsenic. Given the complexity of the treatment and its low efficacy (about a 30% cure rate), many physicians felt the treatment was worse than the disease.

Yet, with the assistance of the U.S. Public Health Service, this effort achieved some success. In 1930, however, Rosenwald funding was discontinued following the 1929 stock market crash. With this source of funding gone, the Public Health Service (PHS) decided to limit its efforts to a small research project: the PHS staff would follow a group of untreated men for 6 to 8 months, then administer treatment. The senior PHS officer assigned to the project, Dr. Taliaferro Clark, was one of a group of PHS syphilologists who were considered liberal on racial matters in that they had some concern for the health of African Americans. Yet he wrote to a colleague, "These negroes are very ignorant and easily influenced by things that would be of minor significance in a more intelligent group" (Brody, 2002).

In 1933, Clark retired and was succeeded by his deputy, Dr. Raymond Vonderlehr. Fascinated by the pathology he was seeing in the men, Vonderlehr developed a plan to offer them partial treatment in order to keep them in the study. At this point, the project became a long-term study of untreated—actually undertreated—syphilis. It was Vanderlehr and his colleague, Dr. Oliver Wenger, who devised most of the study's deceptive strategies to ensure the cooperation of the subjects. Writing to Vanderlehr regarding his tactic of calling spinal taps (often-painful diagnostic tests used to detect neurosyphilis) a "free special treatment," Wenger congratulated him on his "flair for framing letters to Negroes." Clark also defended this tactic (Brody, 2002).

The study initially included 300 men with syphilis and 300 without. Early in the project, 99 of the controls developed syphilis and were moved into the experimental group.

Although the project was devised and led by the White leaders of the Venereal Disease Section of the USPHS, it could not have succeeded without the cooperation and support of local Black leadership. Moton agreed to support the study if "Tuskegee gets its full share of the credit" and if Black professionals were involved. The latter condition was met by the inclusion of Dr. Eugene Dibble, head of Tuskegee Institute's John Andrews Hospital. He supported the institute's full cooperation and involvement in the study, which he wrote in a letter to Moton would "offer very valuable training for our students as well as for the interns . . . our own hospital and the Tuskegee Institute would get credit for this piece of research work" (Brody, 2002).

Even more important to the study was nurse Eunice Rivers, who was working at John Andrews Hospital in 1931 and who was recommended to the study's directors by Eugene Dibble. Rivers was responsible for the project's outreach efforts, contacting the men in their homes, explaining their disease to them, informing them about the project, and often driving them to the study's clinical facilities. In many ways, she was a "culturally competent" public health nurse. Rivers was the only person to work in the project for the entirety of its 40-year duration.

The role of these and other Black professionals in the Tuskegee Syphilis Study has been the subject of much discussion and will be further considered later in this chapter.

At no time was the Tuskegee Syphilis Study conducted in secret. To the contrary, it was well known throughout the Public Health Service and it generated numerous scientific papers in the medical literature. The first of these appeared in 1936 (Vonderlehr, Clark, Wenger, &

Heller). At least 22 other publications followed (see Appendix) as well as numerous lectures, presentations at scientific meetings, and unpublished reports. Hence, for 40 years the project was conducted in full view of the scientific community, with little or no question raised regarding its ethics.

Preventing the men from being treated sometimes required unusual efforts. The World War II draft represented one such challenge, because many of the study's subjects were at risk of being drafted and treated by the Army. However, standing in the way of treatment was in some respects defensible, because as previously noted, the treatment was toxic and of limited effectiveness.

That changed radically in 1945, however. Penicillin had emerged as an effective and safe treatment for syphilis. With the end of the war, it became readily available. By 1947, the PHS had established Rapid Treatment Centers as part of a national program of syphilis control, and U.S. case rates subsequently declined dramatically. In Tuskegee, however, the subjects of the Tuskegee Syphilis Study continued to go untreated. The cooperation of local physicians was now more crucial than ever, because it was not only essential to withhold treatment for the men's syphilis, but also to withhold treatment for other infections because the penicillin used might concurrently treat the syphilis. Hence, the subjects of the study, without their consent, were put at risk for a variety of other infectious diseases in addition to syphilis.

In 1947 a program of rotating African American medical students through the study unit was also initiated. By 1962, 127 such students had been rotated through the unit. This represented another way in which the study was exposed to scrutiny without repercussion.

In the late 1960s, questions regarding the ethics of the study were raised in *The Drum*, a civil rights newsletter published by employees of the Department of Health, Education, and Welfare [HEW]. In 1966, Peter Buxtun, a PHS venereal disease investigator in San Francisco, read about the study and wrote a letter to the Public Health Service's National Communicable Disease Center (NCDC; now the Centers for Disease Control and Prevention, or CDC) where the study was housed, challenging its ethics. Although ignored initially, Buxtun persisted, and his persistence resulted in the creation of a blue-ribbon committee by the NCDC director to review the study and recommend whether it should be continued (Jones, 1993).

The committee reported in the affirmative: the study should indeed be continued. In fact, in the committee's view, it was important at that point in time to strengthen the study and to enlist additional local support for it. Endorsements were subsequently sought and obtained from the Alabama State Health Department, the Macon County Health Department, and the Macon County Medical Society, which was predominantly Black.

Hence, the study continued, alive and well, until 1972. Peter Buxtun had by then left the PHS to enroll in law school. Eventually he described the Tuskegee Syphilis Study to a newspaper reporter friend who worked for the Associated Press. The story was assigned to another reporter, Jean Heller, who broke the story in the *Washington Star* on July 25, 1972. The next day, Dr. Merlin Duval, HEW's assistant secretary for health, told reporters that he was "shocked and horrified" by the Tuskegee Syphilis Study (Jones, 1993).

And that ended the study. Eventually, the syphilitic men who were still alive were treated for their disease as appropriate and also guaranteed free medical care for the remainder of their lives. A $1.8 billion lawsuit filed by civil rights attorney Fred Gray was settled out of court in 1974 for $10 million (Reverby, 1997) and the money was divided among more than 600 survivors, spouses, and descendants of the study's original subjects.

On May 16, 1997, the five remaining Tuskegee survivors who were able to make the trip flew to Washington to receive a personal apology from President Clinton. In his remarks at the time, the president said, "The United States government did something that was wrong—deeply, profoundly, morally wrong. It was an outrage to our commitment to integrity and equality for all our citizens . . . I am sorry that your federal government orchestrated a study so clearly racist" (Clinton, 1997).

Although the Tuskegee Syphilis Study ended more than three decades ago, it has continued to have profound implications for the way in which research on human participants is conducted in this country and has special implications for community-based research in African American communities.

CHANGED RESEARCH PRACTICES SINCE 1972

In 1974, in the aftermath of the scandal surrounding the Tuskegee Syphilis Study, the National Research Act was signed into law, creating the National Commission for the Protection of Human Subjects of Biomedical and Behavioral Research (National Commission). In 1979, the commission issued the Belmont Report, which articulated a set of ethical principles that continue to guide human research in the U.S. (National Commission, 1979). It must be noted, however, that the commission did not invent research ethics. Well-known ethical codes for research that antedated it include the Nuremberg Code (Mitscherlich & Mielke, 1949) and the Declaration of Helsinki (World Medical Association, 1964). Both demanded that research on humans be carried out only with the informed consent of the subjects.

The ethical principles, as stated in the Belmont Report (National Commission, 1974) are as follows:

1. *Respect for Persons.* Respect for persons incorporates at least two ethical convictions: first, that individuals should be treated as autonomous agents, and second, that persons with diminished autonomy are entitled to protection. The principle of respect for persons thus divides into two separate moral requirements: the requirement to acknowledge autonomy and the requirement to protect those with diminished autonomy.

2. *Beneficence.* Persons are treated in an ethical manner not only by respecting their decisions and protecting them from harm, but also by making efforts to secure their well-being. . . . Two general rules have been formulated as complementary expressions of beneficent actions in this sense: (1) do not harm, and (2) maximize possible benefits and minimize possible harms. [This is sometimes expressed as two separate principles: beneficence and nonmaleficence.]

3. *Justice.* Who ought to receive the benefits of research and bear its burdens? This is a question of justice, in the sense of "fairness in distribution" or "what is deserved." An injustice occurs when some benefit to which a person is entitled is denied without good reason or when some burden is imposed unduly.

The Department of Health, Education, and Welfare already had regulations in place governing federally funded research, but these were revised following the publication of the Belmont Report (National Commission, 1979) (45 C.F.R. 46). Simultaneously, the Food and Drug Administration (FDA) revised its regulations (21 C.F.R. 50, 56). The new regulations, like the old ones, focused primarily on properly obtaining informed consent to participate in research. They also required institutions receiving federal research funds to establish ethics committees known as Institutional Review Boards to review each research proposal involving human subjects to determine whether it met ethical standards. In addition, the regulations established requirements for confidentiality for persons participating in research.

In 1991, 16 federal departments and agencies (later expanded to 18) became signatories to 45 C.F.R. 46, and its core (Subpart A) became known as the Common Rule. However, some federal agencies that conduct human research are not covered by the Common Rule, and the FDA continues to have additional regulations that cover research on drugs and devices (National Bioethics Advisory Commission, 2001).

Despite the additional safeguards put in place by the new regulations, however, knowledge of the Tuskegee Syphilis Study continues to foster a deep suspicion of research in the African American community. As stated by Gamble (1997a), "since its public revelation, the study has moved from a singular historical event to a powerful metaphor that symbolizes racism in medicine, misconduct in human research, the arrogance of physicians, and government abuse of black people." Distrust of the biomedical community generally and of researchers in particular is especially visible when research is to be done in the field in an African American community (rather than in a hospital or clinic). Scientists doing such research are unlikely to avoid it for long.

DISCUSSION

Four issues deserve further discussion: (a) the study's specific ethical violations; (b) the question of how reputable scientists could participate in and defend the project; (c) the role of African Americans in the study; and (d) contemporary racism in the United States.

Ethical Violations

As described earlier, the Belmont Report defined three ethical principles: respect for persons, beneficence, and justice. The Tuskegee Syphilis Study violated all three.

Respect for persons is synonymous with *autonomy*. This is every person's right to act as an independent agent, free of coercion and armed with the facts. By failing to explain the study to the men who were its subjects—and worse, by deceiving them into thinking that they were receiving treatment rather than serving as the subjects of research—the Tuskegee Syphilis Study's researchers denied them their autonomy. The researchers frequently rationalized this by stating their belief that the men were too ignorant and poorly educated to understand an explanation or to give truly informed consent. Eventually, this was demonstrated to be false. The men who survived at least until 1972 showed that they were indeed capable of understanding what had been done to them; but if they had not been thus capable, they would have been deserving of special protections, not subject to an arbitrary abrogation of their right to autonomy. The Belmont Report articulated this clearly (National Commission, 1979).

Beneficence is the moral obligation to act for the benefit of others and to promote good. Sometimes its obverse, *nonmaleficence*—the obligation not to inflict harm on others—is stated as a separate ethical principle. This principle clearly is central to the practice of medicine, in which the physician is expected to offer a treatment with known efficacy. If no such treatment is available, the physician should at least be sure not to worsen the patient's condition (according to the Hippocratic maxim, "First, do no harm"). In research, the application of the ethical principle is less obvious, because the efficacy and safety of the treatment under study are unproven. The investigator cannot be certain that the research will benefit the participant, and it may in fact cause harm. As the Belmont Report states, however, "investigators and members of their institutions are obliged to give forethought to the maximization of benefits and the reduction of risk that might occur from the research investigation" (National Commission, 1979). In the Tuskegee Syphilis Study, both parts of the beneficence/nonmaleficence principle were abandoned: treatment was not only withheld by the investigators, but they also attempted to ensure that the men were not treated by other physicians even if it meant that other, nonsyphilitic, infections also went untreated. Hence, there was no attempt to provide any benefit to the subjects and many of the researchers' actions risked a positive harm. Ironically, the only tangible benefit associated with participating in the Tuskegee Syphilis Study was a promise by the government to pay the subjects' funeral expenses.

The third principle, *justice,* calls for fair, equitable, and appropriate treatment in light of what is due or owed to persons. In research, this consideration applies largely to the selection of participants: No one segment of society should bear a disproportionate share of the risks of research; similarly, no one segment should benefit disproportionately. This principle was violated rather routinely during the nineteenth century and the first half of the twentieth, when "the burdens of serving as research subjects fell largely upon poor ward patients, while the benefits of improved medical care flowed primarily to private patients" (National Commission, 1979). The Tuskegee Syphilis Study was but a particularly egregious example of this; only poor, uneducated African Americans were made to assume the risks of the study, although the disease being studied was not confined to that segment of the population. More than any other, the violation of this principle by the Tuskegee Syphilis Study—as well as by many other studies and by the health care establishment generally—has bred mistrust and suspicion in African American and other minority communities.

Participation of Scientists in the Tuskegee Syphilis Study

One of the most fascinating aspects of the Tuskegee history is that it was not carried out in secret by a clandestine group of Nazis, but rather was conducted by leading public health physicians, otherwise ethical men, in full view of the entire medical community. Somehow, a project that was seen as quite acceptable by almost all of the many people who knew about it was reevaluated and became, literally overnight, the embodiment of unethical research. What was everybody thinking?

Several explanations must be considered. One is the tenor of the times, especially during the study's first 30 years. As noted previously, it was commonplace—at least until the Tuskegee Syphilis Study was exposed in the lay press—for research to be carried out on people who were poor with little or no thought given to informed consent. The Tuskegee Syphilis Study was not the only example of this. Another research project that gained considerable notoriety was the Willowbrook Study, carried out from 1963 through 1966 at the Willowbrook State School, an institution for those who were mentally retarded, in Staten Island, New York. There, children were deliberately infected with hepatitis in order to study the infection's natural history and to test the value of gamma globulin in preventing or treating it (University of California, 2000).

In addition, it was an era in which overt, undiluted racism was the norm, especially in southern states such as Alabama. Segregation was based on the premise that Blacks truly were inferior to Whites (intellectually, morally, and socially), and this code was endorsed by most Whites and at least accepted by Blacks, as exemplified by Booker T. Washington's quote at the outset of this chapter. Hence, exploiting

African Americans for the benefit of science would not warrant opprobrium.

Particularly disturbing, then, was the February 6, 1969, meeting that was called at NCDC, after Peter Buxtun persisted in his criticisms, to consider whether the study should be continued. By that time, the Civil Rights movement had made its mark, the last vestiges of de jure segregation were crumbling, and the times had clearly changed. This would seem to have been a great opportunity to admit that errors had been made and to discontinue the project. The committee, all physicians, consisted of three professors, the state health officer from Alabama, and a senior officer from the Milbank Memorial Fund. In addition, several high-ranking PHS officials were in attendance. Only one committee member, Dr. Gene Stollerman of the University of Tennessee, argued for discontinuation of the study on ethical grounds. The others all considered that the study represented a great scientific opportunity and maintained that penicillin treatment might do more harm than good by triggering adverse reactions (Jones, 1993).

It appeared that the motivating force in the room was what might be called the "scientific imperative"—the idea that advancing science was the value that trumped all others and was to be pursued regardless of other considerations. It is now almost universally acknowledged that little or nothing of scientific value was generated by the Tuskegee Syphilis Study.

Scientists are highly motivated to seek self-actualization (perhaps glory) through their work. To complete a major study that results in publications is to achieve a certain type of immortality. Thus, the scientific zeal for this study may be understood even as it crossed ethical boundaries.

The Role of African-Americans in the Study

Perhaps even more perplexing was the collaboration of African American professionals. Robert Moton (the president of Tuskegee Institute), Dr. Eugene Dibble (the head of John Andrews Hospital), nurse Eunice Rivers, the members of the Macon County Medical Society, 127 African American medical students, and others all signed off on the study and some expended considerable effort to support it. In the case of Eunice Rivers, it was virtually her entire career.

Moton, Dibble, and others who approved of the study at the beginning apparently saw it as a way to boost the prestige of Tuskegee Institute as a key participant in an important scientific study. They accepted at face value the importance ascribed to the study by the Public Health Service. This willingness to defer to the experts probably also explains the endorsement of the study by the Macon County Medical Society in 1969. These were, after all, country doctors in the presence of scientists from the National Communicable Disease Center.

Eunice Rivers, who in her role was the very epitome of caring, apparently saw this caring as a form of treatment. She understood that the work she was performing for these very poor men—which included offering them vitamins, aspirin, and iron, finding food for them in the hardest times, and helping them in many other ways—was much more than they would have had if the study had not existed. "These people were given good attention for their particular time," she said in an interview after the study had closed. Moreover, it was not likely that a nurse of Rivers' day would ever have questioned doctor's orders, although she did insist that the PHS physicians treat the men with a modicum of dignity. She said she told the physicians, "Don't mistreat my patients. You don't mistreat them, now, 'cause they don't have to come. And if you mistreat them I will not let them [come] up here to be mistreated" (Reverby, 1997).

Contemporary Racism in the U.S.

Racism remains a pervasive force in America today (Jones, 1993). Although interpersonal forms may seem more benign than in the past, structural, institutionalized racism persists and is still a major determinant of health and health policy. The most deleterious form of racism is subtle and complex because it results in differences in socioeconomic status and interacts with culture and a host of political and other factors. In addition, there are differences in the perception of the existence of racism according to one's personal experiences: according to an ABC News poll in October 2001, 22% of Whites see American society as discriminating against Blacks, while 57% of Blacks view society in that way (Langer, 2001).

The Tuskegee Syphilis Study is by no means the sole reason African Americans are suspicious of researchers and the health care system. The mistrust was prevalent before the study was generally known and has continued despite the new government regulations and the President's apology. It stems from abuses that were a part of slavery, continued through the Jim Crow era, and are seen today in various contemporary manifestations of racism (Byrd & Clayton, 2001; Gamble, 1997b).

CONCLUSIONS

The Tuskegee Study of Untreated Syphilis in the Negro Male started out as an effort to do good, or at least to do good science. It was well managed: It followed 600 men for 40 years with a loss to follow-up of only 17%. It was culturally appropriate; certainly any community-based study would wish for a Nurse Rivers to serve as point person, and offering funeral expenses as an incentive was on target. It involved community institutions, churches, businesses, and physicians (Black and White). And yet it was the most infamous violation of research ethics in American history.

Despite all of the ethical safeguards put in place since 1972, the only real safeguard is an educated community that asks questions about the ethics of interventions and research carried out in the community. The extent to which White Americans want to believe that this study is an aberration is the extent to which they try to absolve themselves from their responsibility. The extent to which Black Americans see this as a conspiracy is the extent to which they seek to absolve themselves of *their* responsibility.

Public health in the South began in the 1930s with the provision of services to poor and Black communities with the goal of protecting the health and welfare of White Southerners. In the 1960s public health began to provide services to poor and Black communities in order to improve the health of those communities. Today, we must find better ways to provide prevention and public health services within our communities, and community-based research is the means by which those better ways can be found. However, there must be community participation in each phase of these research programs—as well as service programs—to achieve the goals of healthy people in healthy communities. The manner in which we seek to close the health status gap is as important as closing the gap itself. Meaningful participation is important and the reader is referred to the *levels of participation* described in chapter 1. To quote Martin Luther King, "If we are to survive today and realize the dream of our mission and the dream of the world, we must bridge the gulf and somehow keep the means by which we live abreast with the ends for which we live" (as cited in Washington, 1986).

RECOMMENDED READINGS
ON THE TUSKEGEE SYPHILIS STUDY

Brant, A. M. (1978). *Racism and research: The case of the Tuskegee syphilis study.* Hastings Center Report.

Department of Health, Education, and Welfare, Public Health Service. (1973). *Final report of the Tuskegee syphilis study.* Ad hoc Advisory Panel.

Jones, J. H. (1993). *Bad blood: The Tuskegee syphilis experiment.* New York: The Free Press.

Reverby, S. (2000). *Tuskegee's truths: Rethinking the Tuskegee syphilis study.* Chapel Hill: University of North Carolina Press.

White, R. M. (2000). Unraveling the Tuskegee study of untreated syphilis. *Archives of Internal Medicine, 160,* 585–598.

APPENDIX

Chronological Bibliography of Papers Written While the Tuskegee Syphilis Study Was Being Conducted

Vondelehr, R. A. Circa 1934. Introduction to the Tuskegee study. Unpublished.

Vonderlehr, R. A., Clark, T., Wenger, O. C., & Heller, J. R. (1936). Untreated syphilis in the male negro. *Journal of Venereal Disease Information, 17,* 260–265.

Parran, T. (1937). Control of syphilis: Clinical lecture at Atlantic City session. Unknown publication.

Clark, Taliaferro, Wenger, Oliver, Vondelehr, R. A., Heller, J. R., et al. Circa 1938. *History and background of study of untreated syphilis in the male negro in Macon County, Alabama.* Unpublished.

Sowder, W. T. (1940). An interpretation of Bruusgaard's paper on the fate of untreated syphilitics. *American Journal of Syphilis, Gonorrhea, and Venereal Disease, 24,* 684–691.

Deibert, A. V., & Bruyere, M. C. (1946). Untreated syphilis in the male negro III. Evidence of cardiovascular abnormalities and other forms of morbidity. *Journal of Venereal Diseases Information,* 301–314.

Heller, J. R., & Bruyere, P. T. (1946). Untreated syphilis in the male negro II. Mortality during 12 years of observation. *Journal of Venereal Disease Information,* 34–38.

Usilton, L. J., & Miner, J. R. (1946). A tentative death curve for acquired syphilis in white and colored males in the United States. *Journal of Venereal Disease Information, 18,* 231–239.

Rosahn, P. D. (1946). Studies in syphilis VII. The end results of untreated syphilis. *Journal of Venereal Disease Information,* 293–301.

Unknown Author. Circa 1948. *Serologic evaluation of patients included in the Tuskegee study.* Unpublished.

Unknown Author. (Circa 1949). Tuskegee autopsy study. Unpublished manuscript.

Pesere, P. J., Bauer, T. J., & Gleeson, G. A. (1950). Untreated syphilis in the male negro: Observation of abnormalities over sixteen years. *American Journal of Syphilis, Gonorrhea, and Venereal Diseases, 34,* 201–213.

Unknown Author. (1952). *Gross pathological changes found at postmortem examinations in untreated syphilitics.* Unpublished.

Olansky, S., Simpson, L., & Schuman, S. (1954). Untreated syphilis in the male negro: Environmental factors in the Tuskegee study of untreated syphilis. *Public Health Reports, 69,* 691–698.

Shafer, J. K., Usilton, L. J., & Gleeson, G. A. (1954). Untreated syphilis in the male negro: A prospective study of the effect on life expectancy. *Milbank Memorial Fund Quarterly,* 262–274.

Smith, C. A., et. al. (1955). *Untreated syphilis in the male negro.* U.S. Public Health Service. Unpublished Manuscript.

Schuman, S. H., Olansky, S., Rivers, E., Smith, C. A., & Rambo, D. S. (1955). Untreated syphilis in the male negro: Background and current status of patients in the Tuskegee study. *Journal of Chronic Disease, 2,* 543–558.

Peters, J. J., Peers, J. H., Olansky, S., Cutler, J. C., & Gleeson, G. A. (1955). Untreated syphilis in the male negro: Pathologic findings in syphilitic and nonsyphilitic patients. *Journal of Chronic Disease,* 127–148.

Olansky, S., Harris, A., Cutler, J. C., & Price, E. V. (1956). Untreated syphilis in the male negro: Twenty-two years of serologic observation in a syphilis study group. *A.M.A. Archives of Dermatology,* 516–522.

Olansky, S., Schuman, S., Peters, J., Smith, C. A., & Rambo, D. S. (1956). Untreated syphilis in the male negro: Twenty two years of clinical observation of untreated syphilitic and presumably nonsyphilitic groups. *Journal of Chronic Disease,* 177–185.

Rivers, E., Schuman, S. H., Simpson, L., & Olansky, S. (1963). Twenty years of follow-up experience in a long range medical study. *Public Health Reports, 68,* 391–395.

Rockwell, D. H., Yobs, A. R., & Moore, M. B. (1964). The Tuskegee study of untreated syphilis: The 30th year of observation. *Archives of Internal Medicine, 114,* 792–798.

Background Paper on Tuskegee study. (1972). Venereal Disease Branch, State and Community Services Division, Center for Disease Control.

Goldwater, L. J. (1973). The Tuskegee study in historical perspective. Unpublished typescript. *The Lancet,* 1438.

Caldwell, J. G., Price, E. V., & Schroeter, A. L. (1973). Aortic regurgitation in the Tuskegee study of untreated syphilis. *Journal of Chronic Disease, 26,* 187–194.

REFERENCES

Brody, H. (2002). *Faces of Tuskegee.* Retrieved from Michigan State University Web site HM546 Ethics Module: http://www.msu.edu/course/hm/546/tuskegee.htm

Brunner, B. (2000). *The Tuskegee syphilis experiment: The U.S. government's 40-year experiment on black men with syphilis.* http://www.infoplease.com/spot/bhmtuskegee1.html

Byrd, W. M., & Clayton, L. A. (2001). *An American health dilemma: Race, medicine, and health care in the United States.* New York: Routledge.

Centers for Disease Control. Tuskegee Syphilis Study Page. http://www.cdc.gov/nchstp/od/tuskegee/

Clinton, W. (1997, May 16). Remarks by the President in apology for study done in Tuskegee. The White House, Office of the Press Secretary. Available at: http://clinton4.nara.gov/textonly/New/Remarks/Fri/19970516-898.html

Gamble, V. N. (1997a, Fall). The Tuskegee syphilis study and women's health. *Journal of American Medical Womens Association, 52,* 195–196.

Gamble, V. N. (1997b). Under the shadow of Tuskegee: African Americans and health care. *American Journal of Public Health, 87*(11), 1773–1778.

Jones, J. H. (1993). *Bad blood: The Tuskegee syphilis experiment.* New York: The Free Press.

Langer, G. (n.d.). *Most see racial discrimination.* http://abcnews.go.com/sections/politics/DailyNews/poll991025.html

Mitscherlich, A., & Mielke, F. (Eds.). (1947). *Doctors of infamy: The story of the Nazi medical crimes.* New York: Schuman.

Moton, R. R. (1921). *Finding a way out: An autobiography.* Garden City, NY: Doubleday, Page. Full text available at University of North Carolina Web site: http://docsouth.unc.edu/moton/menu.html

National Bioethics Advisory Commission. (2001, August). *Ethical and policy issues in research involving human participants.* Bethesda MD. Available at http://bioethics.georgetown.edu/nbac/human/overvol1.pdf

National Commission for the Protection of Human Subjects of Biomedical and Behavioral Research. (1979). *The Belmont report: Ethical principles and guidelines for the protection of human subjects of research.* Bethesda, MD: National Institutes of Health. Available at http://ohrp.osophs.dhhs.gov/humansubjects/guidance/belmont.htm

Reverby, S. (1997). History of an apology: From Tuskegee to the White House [Electric version]. *Research Nurse, 3*(4). http://www.researchpractice.com/archive/apology.shtml

University of California at Santa Barbara. Human Subjects Training Module. (2000). Retrieved from *Willowbrook hepatitis study.* http://hstraining.orda.ucsb.edu/training/willowbrook.htm

Vonderlehr, R. A., Clark, T., Wenger, O. C., & Heller, J. R. (1936). Untreated syphilis in the male negro. *Journal of Venereal Disease Information, 17,* 260–265.

Washington, J. M. (Ed.). (1986). *A Testament of Hope: The Essential Writings of Martin Luther King, Jr.* New York: Harper Collins.

World Medical Association. (1964, June). *Declaration of Helsinki.* Adopted by the 18th World Medical Assembly, Helsinki, Finland. Available at: http://ohsr.od.nih.gov/helsinki.php3

Chapter 4

THE VIEW FROM THE COMMUNITY

*Andrea Cruz, Fred Murphy, Nana Nyarko,
and D. N. Yung Krall*

We argued in chapter 1 that researchers should create partnerships with communities and be guided by what communities have to say. Further, researchers must understand that community perspectives and the language in which those perspectives are expressed are likely to differ from those of scholars and academics. We have applied that philosophy to editing this book by soliciting community contributions, and those contributions are offered in this chapter.

Some references were supplied by the contributors; we have added some others to indicate support in the scientific literature for some of the assertions made. What is not referenced may be considered to be the view of the author.

At least some of what is discussed in one section of the chapter may be applicable to other sections as well. For instance, the discussion of community empowerment and community ownership in the section on the African American community would be equally appropriate in either of the other sections.

—*The Editors*

THE HISPANIC COMMUNITY

The most rapidly growing minority in the United States includes Mexicans, Chicanos, Puerto Ricans, Cubans, Dominicans, Colombians, and Salvadorians, all of whom are labeled Latino or Hispanic. The terms include many different cultural values, beliefs, and religious backgrounds, just as Latin America includes many countries and many diverse peoples.

There are approximately 32.4 million Hispanics living in the United States. By the year 2005, Hispanics will be the largest minority population in the country. Moreover, between 2000 and 2050, Hispanics will account for the majority of the nation's population growth (U.S. Census, 2000).

Differences among Hispanics are influenced by

- education
- socioeconomic status
- immigration status
- age
- length of time in the United States
- degree to which they have adopted Anglo behavior and values
- rural versus urban residence
- country of origin, or of ancestral origin, including experiences there

Because of these differences, many Latinos (referring to the region of origin, Latin America, which includes many countries) prefer to be called Hispanic (referring to the common language, Spanish). Among the diverse Hispanic population, there exists considerable ethnocentrism (Huddy & Virtanen, 1995). Conflicts among the groups are common, and distinctions may be made on the basis of nationality, class, or other characteristics. Although Hispanics share strong family values, class-based differences are apparent. Distinctions are drawn along the lines of lower, middle, or upper class, as well as along the lines of blue collar versus professional worker, legal versus undocumented immigrant, and English speakers versus non-English-speakers. Whatever one's circumstances are, there is a label and a corresponding potential for discrimination by those under other circumstances.

Hispanic families are usually very extended (Blank & Torrechila, 1998). Members include in-laws, godparents, and in many cases, long-time friends and neighbors. During a crisis, a family usually comes together. It is not unusual to discover that half of the community has gathered for support. Hispanic families live in clusters, and often in subclusters, especially among Mexicans. A cluster may consist of people who come from the state of Oaxaca, Hidalgo, Guerrero, or Puebla. Many people from rural areas speak Spanish only as a second language and replicate their village as they relocate to the United States.

Nonverbal communication is commonly practiced by Hispanics (Rodriguez, 1999). This may cause confusion and even physical punishment when dealing with non-Hispanics who are not aware of important nonverbal cues. For instance, Hispanic parents teach their children to look down as a sign of respect when dealing with adults. Anglo schoolteachers, however, generally expect eye contact to ensure understanding.

Respect and manners are considered the most important part of family values. Elderly family members receive much respect and protection (Williams, Tappen, Buscemi, Rivera, & Lezcano, 2001). Family members care for their elders, including elderly members of the extended family. It is considered a lack of respect to ignore or avoid giving support to the family in time of a crisis. Hispanics tend to be very private. It takes more than a good interpreter to convince them to share personal information. This may seriously impair communication with health care professionals.

Health and Health Care in the Hispanic Community

Home remedies are prevalent, and many Hispanics believe strongly in herbs and other drugs sold in their home countries (Bonkowsky, Frazer, Buchi, & Byington, 2002; Keegan, 1996). Though antibiotics are prescription drugs in the U.S., they are easily obtained without a prescription in Mexico and other Latin American countries. Frequently Hispanics will bring drugs back from their home country for personal use or for resale in the States. This represents a law-enforcement issue, and as a consequence, Hispanics often withhold information about black-market antibiotic use from their physicians. Moreover, it is commonly believed that an injection is more effective than an oral drug, and it is often expected that a physician will supply one (McVea, 1997). This is less likely if the physician recognizes that the patient is already taking an oral antibiotic.

Removing blood is very worrisome, particularly to less-educated Hispanic immigrants from rural villages. Blood is a sacred substance, the liquid of life. Its removal should not be taken lightly. Rarely will Hispanics participate in blood drives. Hispanics commonly become hesitant when lab work is to be done, whether for treatment or research purposes. They will ask why they must have blood drawn. The response to this question should be more than the usual "informed consent." This is true for other more intimate or private forms of examination as well. It is often effective to engage in an initial period of friendly, informal conversation before discussing serious issues such as these; this helps to avoid appearing unfriendly or discourteous and allows the establishment of trust and support.

Their limited use and understanding of English is frustrating to those who do not speak this language well. However, typically they do not react well to criticism. In Hispanic men, frustration often leads to domestic violence (Lown & Vega, 2001). The language barrier prevents them from becoming confrontational with those outside the community—those with whom they are experiencing frustration—but they may instead become hostile and violent with a spouse or family member. Domestic violence is a silent problem in the Hispanic community. Women are kept in isolation to protect family secrets, while husbands are on the "front lines." Alcoholism may also play a role and may be a coping mechanism for stress and frustration (Caetano, Nelson, & Cunradi, 2001).

Stresses other than the language barrier may include a lack of steady employment, illegal immigration status, and family separation. Families are commonly split while spouses or parents come to the U.S. to work for higher wages than are offered in their home countries. Anglo communities often do not understand why there are 14-, 15-, or 16-year-old Hispanic farmworkers in this country without adult supervision. These teenagers are the main breadwinners for the family left behind. With little or no education, these youngsters are very attractive to employers who seek strong, able-bodied labor for vegetable or fruit harvesting and construction work. The youngsters are warned in advance about the minimum working age in the U.S., so they lie about their age to gain employment opportunities.

It is difficult to obtain steady employment for those who lack English skills and are unskilled. The majority of the Hispanics who work in rural areas consists of migrant and seasonal farm workers or persons who have been in the fields soon after their arrival here. Few come on an employment visa. A lack of proper documentation by the Immigration and Naturalization Service (INS) hinders the ability of these immigrants to obtain a steady job or even to move freely about the country. Agricultural work is seasonal and unpredictable. Minimum wages are not enough to live on while supporting loved ones in the home country.

Hispanics are proud and prefer to work for a living rather than to seek charity or welfare. Some Anglo communities feel that their jobs are threatened as companies learn more about the outstanding work ethic of Hispanics and hire them because of their hard work and commit-ment to their job. However, this opens the door to exploitation and abuse of illegal workers. Undocumented Hispanics will work under any conditions to make money to support their families back home. Suffer-ing under impossible work conditions while trying to make ends meet both here and at home may lead to alcoholism and substance abuse. Men separated from their wives may engage in sex with other men. This secret among Hispanic males is unlikely to be revealed to health professionals or researchers (Wainburg, 1999), and the consequences may be sexually transmitted diseases as well as alcohol and drug-related diseases, including HIV infection.

Sex role differentiation in the Hispanic community is not the same as other cultures. Women tend to be emotionally expressive, but males do not show their emotions. It is the responsibility of the woman to serve as child caregiver and homemaker and to deal with most domestic issues, including health care. With respect to men, *machismo* has changed little from its traditional character (de Leon Siantz, 1994). Hispanic men are free to have extramarital affairs but women are not, and having multiple partners outside of marriage helps to identify them as "real men." Open discussion of sex topics is considered taboo, especially by women, who tend to be sexually conservative.

According to the Centers for Disease Control (CDC) (2000a), more than 18% of AIDS cases are in Hispanics, and 81% of these are in men. Among Hispanics with AIDS who were born in Mexico, 44% were men who have sex with men and 9% were injecting drug users. Among those born in Puerto Rico, however, 14% were men who have sex with men and 48% were injecting drug users (CDC, 2000b). It may thus be seen that HIV prevention efforts must be appropriately tailored for each Hispanic population.

Counseling services are rarely used among Hispanics because of the belief that the system is culturally insensitive (Peifer, Hu, & Vega, 2000). Counseling services appear to Hispanics to be organized and operated to serve middle-class Anglos. Spanish-speaking counselors or therapists are rare. Rather than seek counseling through the health care system, Hispanics are more likely to visit Catholic priests, who are thought to be most appropriate in dealing with issues that are viewed as the work of the Devil.

In the Hispanic family, elderly members are often the family thera-pists. They are perceived as wise, and with wisdom comes knowledge, truth, and respect. Family members and extended family and friends also are sources of counseling. Hispanics also rely on folk healers for many emotional problems, because these healers are perceived as more effective than mental-health workers. There are a variety of such healers in the Hispanic community; they include *curanderos*, who use prayers and artifacts, *yerberos* (herbalists), *espirituistas* (practitioners of spiritualism), and *santeros*, or practitioners of Santeria, who heal through the use of religious artifacts. Relying on these traditional healers is consistent with the common belief that illness has its roots in supernatural forces that include God's will, magical powers, evil spirits, powerful human forces, or emotional upsets. Traditional healers are often viewed with more confidence than are physicians and may be used until illness becomes very severe (Padilla, Gomez, Biggerstaff, & Mehler, 2001). In addition, older family members may offer home remedies (Risser & Mazur, 1995). Diabetes, hypertension, and other serious health problems may be treated with teas, homemade ointments, massages, talismans, or other remedies in which the family believes.

Elderly persons play a special part in family life. It is considered a disgrace to admit one's elderly parents to a nursing home (Williams et al., 2001). Their role in the family is to help in the rearing of grandchildren. In the Hispanic family, children do not traditionally move away at the age of 18; rather, they continue to live at home or near their parents. This is not viewed as dependency, but rather as a support system. Children are expected to follow in their parents' footsteps, and many times they do. They are also expected to seek their parent's advice on important issues.

Hispanics tend to be more concerned about the present than the past or the future, because so many lead a hand-to-mouth existence. Work is the first priority and overshadows family needs. If the child needs immunizations, is sick with a cold, or should be accompanied to school for a teacher conference, this need is secondary to work. A day without work is a week without bread. It thus becomes the responsibility of agencies that provide outreach workers to help to ensure that these needs are met.

Those family providers who are heavily invested in caring for their loved ones tend to acquire a reputation for being late to scheduled appointments. This is sometimes known as "Latin time." Some service organizations that deliver services to Hispanic communities have taken to telling clients that their appointment is a half hour earlier than actually scheduled, hoping that it will result in the client's being on time. The reasons for this chronic tardiness include transportation problems, language barriers, and cultural factors.

Most medical facilities do not provide medical interpreters, and this is often viewed as an act of discrimination and makes their services especially unattractive to non-English-speaking Hispanics (Rollins, 2002). Consequently, Hispanics (as well as other minority groups) are likely to access health care through hospital emergency rooms.

Special Considerations for Community-Based Research in the Hispanic Community

Community-level work among Hispanics requires that one first become acquainted with the community. The researcher should make a few home visits, enjoy the taco she is offered, ignore any housekeeping imperfections, and let the baby put a cookie on her pants. The point is to make people feel comfortable before asking them to participate in a research project.

Survey research requires a good understanding of the educational level and language capabilities of potential participants. Educational levels among migrant and seasonal farmworkers are generally below sixth grade and survey questions should reflect a literacy level that is consistent with this level of education. Never assume that a participant can read.

Questions on sensitive topics should be relatively indirect. For instance, instead of asking, "Do you check your breasts?" consider asking, "Do you know how to do a breast self-exam?" Similarly, instead of asking "Do you use condoms when you have sex?" ask "Do you protect yourself from sexually transmitted diseases when you have relations with someone?" These and other sensitive questions on topics such as domestic violence and drug abuse will elicit responses if asked correctly.

It is important to take into account the priorities of participants, especially those of women. The first priority for a woman is likely to be preparing dinner for her husband. However, survey questions can be asked while the woman works, especially if the surveyor volunteers to care for a child at the same time.

Single males especially are likely to use aliases because of the belief that all documents are accessible to the INS. Clearly, confidentiality is especially important for undocumented persons.

THE AFRICAN AMERICAN COMMUNITY

This section will address three sets of issues that affect approaches to conducting research in African American communities. They include emerging African American perspectives on (a) the meaning of health, (b) community and ways in which researchers can engage it, and (c) complementary and alternative medicine.

Holistic Health

The holistic (or wholistic) approach to health and health care is of increasing interest in the African American community. To be "whole" involves every aspect of life (i.e., body, mind, spirit, and environment) that affects an individual or a community. It is what causes or determines good or bad health. Can an individual live a quality life when any part of the whole is unhealthy?

This question is not a recent one; it emerges from health and temperance reform that has been espoused for decades. As early as the 1800s, educators and scholars were attesting to the relationship between good health and an overall sense of well-being.

In the African American community, such thinking drives the development of concepts such as community ownership, community empowerment, community capacity-building, community development, and community partnerships, among a litany of terms frequently used by health and academic professionals, funding agencies, and policy makers. However, the use of these terms by those in academic or official positions often signifies attention to politically correct wording rather than a real change in how they view health.

What has clearly *not* changed is the traditional structure of American medicine, which, much like an industrial assembly plant is designed for control and to produce standardized practices and outcomes. Under this traditional structure, there are *health care consumers*, a term that has been created over the past two decades or so. Before then, most people could not have imagined being consumers or clients because health was considered a condition, not a commodity.

The traditional approach to health and health care also carries the assumption that what is important about a person, community, or culture is the disease, deficiency, injury, or need. The capacities, competencies, and resources of communities are many times ignored.

For example, a local health agency or institution may determine that diabetes is a serious problem in a particular low-income African American community. It decides to develop and implement a health intervention program to reduce the high prevalence of diabetes in that community. Focus groups are conducted and community meetings arranged at which diabetes and its causes are discussed. This is followed in a few weeks by the announcement of a new community-wide diabetes risk-reduction program. Community residents are encouraged to participate in the program, in a manner that makes the program appear community owned. Unfortunately, however, citizen participation in the new program is low, and the health agency ultimately decides to terminate what it had considered to be a well-thought out, well-designed, and well-intended health intervention program.

What went wrong with this intervention? Diabetes may not have been a priority for this community. Perhaps in the view of the community the most important issue was a problem with sewage disposal, rodent control, or substandard housing—all representing health (but not medical) issues. In this example, the community was deemed by health professionals to be a group of consumers or clients in need of intervention, rather than citizens and community residents capable of determining their own priorities and solutions (Murphy, Satterfield, Anderson, & Lyons, 1993).

A True Community-Ownership Approach

Wallerstein (1992) defines an empowered community as "the associative, self-generated gathering of common people who have sufficient resources in their lives to cope with life's demands and not suffer ill health." In this sense, community-owned health programs focus on the community and cultural capacity (i.e., mental, physical, spiritual, and environmental) of local citizens working as partners with health and academic professions. These programs should be inclusive in nature and be based on community and cultural assets, which shifts the mindset of all involved from one of service-providing to that of capacity-building (true empowerment). Inherent in this shift is the move away from professional domination of providing preventive health programs and care.

There are several implications of this approach for communities as well as for health professionals:

• Agencies and academic institutions must formulate mechanisms for sharing monetary resources with communities through subcontracts or grants to local organizations. These will be accompanied appropriately by accountability for measurable outcomes to which communities must adhere in the short and long run.

- Professionals must respect the historical wisdom of communities concerning their own needs. In most cases, the health professional or researcher is not a part of the community and therefore should open the research project or intervention to permit community residents to have input at each step of the way.
- Community residents must respect the knowledge, information, and infrastructure accessible to health professionals, and allow them to serve as technical facilitators for the project or intervention, as well as fiduciaries between funders and the community.
- Though health professionals and academics can provide information that can help to mobilize communities, they are not the "unit of analysis" in research or the primary source of solutions for community health problems and should therefore proceed with caution in their approach.
- Community residents, on the other hand, are the unit of analysis and the primary source of solutions. They can and should provide insight into the resources and ecology of human behavior within their communities that could not otherwise be discovered by the outside health professional.
- Professionals should use their capabilities, skills, contacts, and resources to conduct training for local leaders and associations, as well as to identify and recognize existing community assets that may be hidden.

The realization that health care, preventive or otherwise, can only be effective if it incorporates into the process those individuals it is seeking to keep well is challenging for many reasons. It is most important that the roles of residents and health professionals be redefined. Both face years of reconditioning. For example, residents must also become nontraditional about their way of living and believe in, and gain insight into, new ways of caring for their health. This will call for them to display wisdom in how they use the resources of their community, and to convince health professionals that they possess the capacity to use and develop the resources.

The consequences of this role awareness will mean that many traditional beliefs, on both sides, will be challenged. However, health professionals and community residents working together can drive changes in the public health mainstream that will improve the quality of life for community residents.

Community Health Assets

Churches. Churches are an asset universally found in African American communities. A considerable literature now exists that documents the experience of partnering with African American churches and church organizations to conduct community-based research and to mount community-health-promotion interventions in a variety of areas ranging from increasing breast cancer screening to improving diet to controlling hypertension (Demark-Wahnefried et al., 2000; Duan, Fox, DeRose, & Carson, 2000; Lewis & Green, 2000; Ofili, Igho-Pemu, & Bransford, 1999; Resnikow et al., 2001; Stockdale, Keeler, Duan, De-Rose, & Fox, 2000; Wilson, 2000). Church-based settings provide opportunities to reach individuals at high risk for disease who would not be reached by traditional means.

Traditional Networks. The network of peers and family members that traditionally provides intimate and confidential health information has been found to have the strongest influence on individuals, especially regarding the safety and good sense of a recommended novel approach to lifestyle and health (Rogers, 1983). Such traditional networks can clearly create barriers to behavior change; however, they also can be activated to promote the adoption of new and beneficial health practices and are thus a potentially important resource.

Opinion Leaders. Credible recognized leaders (opinion leaders) may become effective communicators of health messages to the community and can also serve as informal health educators within the peer network, especially when acting from a basis of shared attributes such as having a high risk of a particular disease. For instance, this approach was shown to be useful in a community intervention trial of an HIV/AIDS prevention intervention among low-income women in housing projects in five U.S. cities (Sikkema et al., 2000).

Community Health Workers. Another approach to bridging the gap between researcher and community is through community health workers (CHWs), also known as lay health workers, community health advisors, and a variety of other titles. There are many published studies documenting the experiences and evaluating the outcomes of training and utilizing community health workers (CDC, 1994a, 1994b), who then become community assets in conducting research, mounting prevention programs, and utilizing other community resources. CHWs have been extensively employed in African American communities. These trained workers can disseminate health information and foster behavior change among individuals at high risk. Their broad-based social support for behavior change can increase the likelihood of adoption and maintenance of the prescribed behaviors (CDC, 1994a, 1994b).

Community Organizations. Community organizations, both formal and informal, provide the arena for social networks that respond to the individual as well as collective needs of the people. Health promotion programs that increase the capacity of existing organizations to deliver legitimate health information and guidance have a greater reach within the target community.

Alternative Approaches to Better Health for Communities

Interest in complementary and alternative medicine is growing in the African American community. Eisenberg et al. (1998) reported that more than 83 million Americans utilize some form of alternative medicine, from massage to weekly yoga classes, acupuncture, or herbal supplements. In 1997, Americans made some 629 million visits to alternative medicine providers, spending more than $17 billion. In this survey, 33.1% of African Americans were reported to have used some form of alternative medicine; this was less than other ethnic groups. Many health practices that are regarded as alternative medicine in the United States by medical care professions are considered traditional medicine in other countries. The effective combination of traditional U.S. medicine and alternative or unconventional medicines has been recently termed "integrative medicine" (Editorial, 1998) and has as its goal treating the whole person, rather than focusing on individual symptoms. Integrative medicine covers a host of therapies and practices, but all share at their core the philosophy of empowering the individual to participate fully in their recovery and maintenance of future health, while emphasizing good nutrition, appropriate exercise, adequate sleep, and stress reduction. Members of the medical community have recognized the need for a more holistic approach to conventional medicine for many years. In 1991, the National Institutes of Health (NIH) established the Office of Alternative Medicine, which serves as a clearinghouse for information on alternative therapies and awards research grants (Harlan, 2001). A number of the nation's medical schools offer courses in integrative medicine (Brokaw, Tunnicliff, Raess, & Saxon, 2002). Insurance companies are under increasing pressure to reassess their coverage of certain therapies (Pelletier & Astin, 2002). Can integrative medicine be a positive and effective public health approach to risk reduction for those population groups at highest risk for disability and disease, such as low-income African Americans? Can it help to improve the health status and subsequently the overall quality of life of those individuals and communities without access to mainstream and high cost medical services?

It is clear that traditional public health and medical care has not worked for the disenfranchised populations of the United States, as evidenced by the disparities in risk, morbidity, and mortality particularly among African Americans as compared to Whites. Health professionals must become more "nontraditional" in their approach to communities and cultures where they are viewed as outsiders.

THE SOUTHEAST ASIAN COMMUNITY

The Asian community is a very diverse one; Chinese, Thai, Vietnamese, Cambodian, Laotian, and people of many other ethnic origins are all labeled Asian in this country. These are groups whose language, food, and customs are all quite different. They share many characteristics, however, and most Southeast Asians have in common the reason they came to the U.S.: They are refugees from the wars and violence that have devastated their homelands for the last 60 years and from the aftermath of those events.

They do not necessarily feel that they are strangers to research, however. For instance, the antibiotic lincomycin was used freely in Vietnam, Thailand and other Southeast Asian countries. When the southeast Asian refugees came to the U.S., their doctors told them that lincomycin has bad side effects and is not used here. Those who had taken it felt sad and angry that they had been used as guinea pigs.

Working in Southeast Asian immigrant communities is, in many ways, like working in other communities. There are informal community leaders in each ethnic community. They could be public health outreach workers, members of a church or temple who are bilingual, or other volunteers in the neighborhoods. Researchers can easily identify them and work with them.

Box 1

When I was a community epidemiologist working with Southeast Asian refugees, my office received a grant to conduct research—a hepatitis B serosurvey—among the refugee population. My boss asked me to be the coordinator and frontline person to deal directly with the refugees and the researchers. I hoped to be able to accept the assignment, but was worried that the research might benefit the researchers but not the refugees. However, in my Vietnamese way, I did not ask her directly "Who is going to benefit from it? And who is paying for it?" I asked: "Will the refugees be vaccinated once we find out if they are good candidates for the vaccine?" My boss assured me that was the main reason for testing thousands of refugees. I was happy then to work on the project.

Southeast Asians are usually willing research participants when they think that the research will help others. Little more is needed than to let people know the roots of the research, explained in clear and simple language (Neufeld, Harrison, Hughes, Spitzer, & Stewart, 2001).

There are boundaries, however. It is not easy to answer strangers' personal questions. Questions concerning family health history are especially taboo in the Southeast Asian community. Southeast Asians are a deeply private people who guard their family's secrets carefully. Often families will keep a child with mental illness or physical deformity out of sight (McKelvey et al., 2002). Though these children are well taken care of, they are not often seen.

Questions that seem acceptable to people of the Western world may be insulting to Southeast Asians. Researchers would do well to ask sensitive questions through skilled interpreters, but must be cautious nonetheless; if questions are asked too sensitively, the responses may be biased as in the example in the next box.

In any event, interviewers should explain sensitive questions before asking them. Asking directly may result in incorrect information or evasions, as in the following question to a married man with STD:

Interviewer: How many sex partners have you had in the last 6 months?
Man: Just my wife.
Interviewer: Then we must test your wife, because you have syphilis.
Man: No, you can't, she and I are separated.

A better approach is to preface the question with a statement such as, "I am going to ask you some very personal questions regarding

---

Box 2

When I spent some time in a family planning clinic in the late 80s, I learned that some of my interpreters took the liberty to skip a few questions that they deemed too intrusive or believed didn't apply to Asian people. One of my Vietnamese clients was a pretty young woman in her late 30s, properly dressed and well-mannered. I asked her many personal and family history medical questions without problems. I had to pause and explain the next question, and asked with a sympathetic look on my face, "How many sexual partners have you had in the last 2 weeks?" The woman looked at me coolly and answered, "Who counts the waves in the ocean?" She was a prostitute and had many medical problems.

Another young client said she was not sexually active and still was a virgin. She was 3 months pregnant. Here I had to be culturally competent to handle the situation, and culturally sensitive not to smile.

---

your health and your lifestyle habits. Your answers will help find better ways to prevent or treat disease." As mentioned previously, Southeast Asians want to be helpful, generally speaking, and will wish to help the researcher or health worker once they understand the nature of the research and the reasons for the questions.

We believe that life is a bittersweet circle and that the good deeds we do today will reward our children or ourselves in the future or in our next life. If we commit bad deeds, however, they will lead to our own or our children's unhappiness. Christians call it "the sin of the father." Buddhists believe in reincarnation. When someone leads a bad life, people may look at that person and say his children will pay for his sin. If a child is born with a congenital defect, neighbors are likely to say that someone in that family must have done something bad that the child must suffer.

Southeast Asian people do not like to be labeled as a minority. In Vietnam, Laos and Cambodia, "minorities" are indigenous tribes who live in the mountains, have little or no contact with outsiders, and who were treated badly by the government, or as primitives. In Vietnam, from time to time, the government would come and give medicine to their children and rock salt to the adults.

In the United States, the term "minority" thus raises concerns. Southeast Asians are proud of their heritage and want to be in mainstream society. They would like to be one of the beautiful threads of the American tapestry and to be known as Vietnamese, Chinese, Laotian, Cambodian, Montagnard, Korean, or Hmong.

There are some additional aspects of Southeast Asian culture in the U.S.:

• Americans may frown at a 16-year-old Laotian bride, but in this culture it is common for young women to marry an older man. She is healthy and will bear healthy babies, while he is older and more established and can support his family.
• In some Vietnamese families, the husband will answer questions for the wife, but in another he may say, "Ask my wife" even in response to questions directed to him.
• Home remedies are common. Generations of Chinese living abroad still use Chinese medicine and home remedies even in their daily diet. Researchers should acknowledge this fact and ask relevant questions with respect.

CONCLUSION

To be effective, the researcher should learn about the characteristics of the targeted community, work with a trusted person in that community, and above all, let people know the purpose of the research. Rejections should not be taken personally.

REFERENCES

Blank, S., & Torrechila, R. S. (1998). Understanding the living arrangements of Latino immigrants: A life course approach. *International Migration Review, 32*, 3–19.

Bonkowsky, J. L., Frazer, J. K., Buchi, K. F., & Byington, C. L. (2000). Metamizole use by Latino immigrants: A common and potentially harmful home remedy. *Pediatrics, 109*, e98.

Brokaw, J. J., Tunnicliff, Raess, B. U., & Saxon, D. W. (2002). The teaching of complementary and alternative medicine in U.S. medical schools: A survey of course directors. *Academic Medicine, 77*, 876–881.

Caetano, R., Nelson, S., & Cunradi, C. (2001). Intimate partner violence, dependence symptoms and social consequences from drinking among white, black and Hispanic couples in the United States. *American Journal of Addiction, 10*(Suppl), 60–69.

Centers for Disease Control. (1994a). Community Health Advisors: Models, Research, and Practice. Selected Annotations—United States. Volume I.

Centers for Disease Control. (1994b). Community Health Advisors:Programs in the United States. Health Promotion and Disease Prevention. Volume II.

Centers for Disease Control. (2000a). HIV/AIDS Surveillance Report. U.S. HIV and AIDS cases reported through December 2000 Year-End Edition Vol. 12, No. 2. Updated Aug 10, 2001 (http://www.cdc.gov/hiv/stats/hasr1202table7.htm)

Centers for Disease Control. (2000b). HIV/AIDS Surveillance Report. U.S. HIV and AIDS cases reported through December 2000 Year-End Edition Vol. 12, No. 2. Updated Aug 10, 2001 (http://www.cdc.gov/hiv/stats/hasr1202/table18.htm#tab19)

de Leon Siantz, M. L. (1994). The Mexican-American migrant farmworker family. Mental health issues. *Nursing Clinics of North America, 29*, 65–72.

Demark-Wahnefried, W., McClelland, J. W., Jackson, B., Campbell, M. K., Cowan, A., Hoben, K., et al. (2000). Partnering with African American churches to achieve better health: lessons learned during the Black Churches United for Better Health 5 a day project. *Journal of Cancer Education, 15*(3), 164–167.

Duan, N., Fox, S. A., Derose, K. P., Carson, S. (2000). Maintaining mammography adherence through telephone counseling in a church-based trial. *American Journal of Public Health, 90*(9), 1468–1471.

Editorial. (1998). *Integrative Medicine, 1*, 1.

Eisenberg, D. M., Davis, R. B., Ettner, S. L., et al. (1998). Trends in alternative medicine use in the United States 1990–1997: Results of a follow-up national survey. *Journal of the American Medical Association, 280*, 1569–1575.

Harlan, W. R., Jr. (2001). Research on complementary and alternative medicine using randomized controlled trials. *Journal of Alternative and Complementary Medicine, 7*(Suppl 1), S45–52.

Huddy, L., & Virtanen, S. (1995). Subgroup differentiation and subgroup bias among Latinos as a function of familiarity and positive distinctiveness. *Journal of Personality and Social Psychology, 68*, 97–108.

Keegan, L. (1996). Use of alternative therapies among Mexican Americans in the Texas Rio Grande Valley. *Journal Holist Nursing, 14*, 277–294.

Lewis, R. K., & Green, B. L. (2000). Assessing the health attitudes, beliefs, and behaviors of African Americans attending church: A comparison from two communities. *Journal of Community Health, 25*(3), 211–224.

Lown, E. A., & Vega, W. A. (2001). Prevalence and predictors of physical partner abuse among Mexican American women. *American Journal of Public Health, 91*, 441–445.

McKelvey, R. S., Sang, D. L., Baldassar, L., Roberts, L., & Cutler, N. (2002). The prevalence of psychiatric disorders among Vietnamese children and adolescents. *Medical Journal of Australia, 21*, 177, 413–417.

McVea, K. L. (1997). Lay injection practices among migrant farmworkers in the age of AIDS: Evolution of a biomedical folk practice. *Social Science and Medicine, 45*, 91–98.

Murphy, F. G., Satterfield, D., Anderson, R. M., & Lyons, A. E. (1993). Diabetes education as cultural translation. *The Diabetes Educator, 19*, 113–115.

Neufeld, A., Harrison, M. J., Hughes, K. D., Spitzer, D., & Stewart, M. J. (2001). Participation of immigrant women family caregivers in qualitative research. *Western Journal of Nursing Research, 23*, 575–591.

Ofili, E., Igho-Pemu, P., & Bransford, T. (1999). The prevention of cardiovascular disease in blacks. *Current Opinion in Cardiology, 14*(2), 169–175.

Padilla, R., Gomez, V., Biggerstaff, S. L., & Mehler, P. S. (2001). Use of curanderismo in a public health care system. *Archives of Internal Medicine, 161,* 1336–1340.

Peifer, K. L., Hu, T., & Vega, W. (2000). Help seeking by persons of Mexican origin with functional impairments. *Psychiatric Services, 51,* 1293–1298.

Pelletier, K. R., & Astin, J. A. (2002). Integration and reimbursement of complementary and alternative medicine by managed care and insurance providers: 2000 update and cohort analysis. *Alternative Therapies in Health and Medicine, 8,* 38–39, 42, 44.

Resnicow, K., Jackson, A., Wang, T., De, A. K., McCarty, F., Dudley, W. N., et al. (2001). A motivational interviewing intervention to increase fruit and vegetable intake through Black churches: Results of the Eat for Life trial. *American Journal of Public Health, 91*(10), 1686–1693.

Risser, A. L., & Mazur, L. J. (1995). Use of folk remedies in a Hispanic population. *Archives of Pediatric and Adolescent Medicine, 149,* 978–981.

Rodriguez, J. (1999). Chaplains' communications with Latino patients: case studies on non-verbal communication. *Journal Pastoral Care, 53,* 309–317.

Rogers, E. M. (1983). *Diffusions of innovations* (3rd ed.). New York: Free Press.

Rollins, G. (2002). Translation, por favor. *Hospital Health Network, 76,* 46–50.

Sikkema, K. J., Kelly, J. A., Winett, R. A., Solomon, L. J., Cargill, V. A., Roffman, R. A., et al. (2000). Outcomes of a randomized community-level HIV prevention intervention for women living in 18 low-income housing developments. *American Journal of Public Health, 90,* 57–63.

Stockdale, S. E., Keeler, E., Duan, N., Derose, K. P., & Fox, S. A. (2000). Costs and cost-effectiveness of a church-based intervention to promote mammography screening. *Health Services Research, 35*(5 Pt 1), 1037–1057.

U.S. Census 2000. www.census.gov/pubinfo/www/hisphot1.html. Accessed August 27, 2003.

Wainberg, M. L. (1999). The Hispanic, gay, lesbian, bisexual and HIV-infected experience in health care. *Mt Sinai Journal of Medicine, 66,* 263–266.

Wallerstein, N. (1992). Powerlessness, empowerment, and health: Implications for health promotion programs. *American Journal of Health Promotion, 6*(3), 197–205.

Williams, C. L., Tappen, R., Buscemi, C., Rivera, R., & Lezcano, J. (2001). Obtaining family consent for participation in Alzheimer's research in a Cuban-American population: Strategies to overcome the barriers. *American Journal of Alzheimers Disease and Other Dementias, 16,* 183–187.

Wilson, L. C. (2000). Implementation and evaluation of church-based health fairs. *Journal of Community Health Nursing, 17*(1), 39–48.

Part II

Methods

Chapter 5

STUDY DESIGNS, SURVEYS, AND DESCRIPTIVE STUDIES

Nabih R. Asal and Laura A. Beebe

GENERAL STUDY DESIGNS

There are two design criteria that serve to delineate three mutually exclusive types of studies: observational, experimental, and quasi-experimental. The first criterion is whether the study factor being investigated is artificially manipulated by the investigator or others. If manipulated, the second criterion is whether categories of the study factor are randomly allocated to all study subjects.

Observational studies are studies involving no artificial manipulation of the study factor. The population is only "observed" with regard to the presence or absence of the study factor(s) or outcome(s). There are two major types of observational studies, *descriptive* and *analytical*. In a descriptive study, the aim is to identify individuals and subgroups who are at high risk and formulate hypotheses for further study. The frequency and distribution of a disease or a health-related state is presented and discussed. In a descriptive study the investigator must identify the characteristics related to person, place, and time. In doing so, the study provides answers to three very important questions: Who is affected by the condition under investigation? Where does a particular health problem occur? and When did it occur? Descriptive studies are usually carried out first in the community and oftentimes provide leads that must be followed up in more refined, controlled analytical studies. The discipline of epidemiology, in its early stages of evolution as a science, relied heavily on descriptive studies of existing mortality and morbidity data sources.

The other major type of observational study is the *analytical study* design. It differs from the descriptive study design in that it requires a comparison group and is a hypothesis-testing method of investigating an association between a study factor and an outcome. There are three primary types of analytical studies:

1. *Cross-sectional (prevalence) study*: The disease or other health outcome and the exposure are measured at one point in time or over a short period of time. Major advantages are that the study is relatively easy to do, does not require a long time to do, and is usually less expensive than other types of analytical studies. It is considered a snapshot of a population. It is an appropriate design to study risk factors for diseases of slow onset but of long duration. However, this study design is limited in that it is not suitable for rare diseases and outcomes or diseases and outcomes of short duration. The sample may not be representative of the population and temporal relationships are difficult to establish. Cross-sectional studies that do not include a comparison group or a hypothesis to be tested are descriptive in nature and do not meet the basic criteria of an analytical study.

2. *Case-control (retrospective) study*: The sampling approach is based on the outcome or disease status. This study design is also called case-referent, or retrospective study. This study begins with identification of an outcome or disease of interest. It identifies subjects with the outcome, called *cases*; and selects subjects for comparison, without the outcome, called *controls*. It looks backward in time (hence the "retrospective" label) to determine what, if any, exposures may have led to the outcome. In other words, the case-control study compares cases with controls with respect to a current or previous study factor.

Case-control studies usually carry the name of the outcome being investigated such as "Case-control Study of Renal Cell Carcinoma, Obesity, and Nutrition" or "Case-control Study of Chronic Renal Disease and Hydrocarbon Exposure." Because a case-control study starts by selecting persons who have the condition of interest, it is useful to study rare diseases. Matching of individual cases and controls (pair match) or groups of cases and controls (frequency match) is often used. The measure of risk and association are the prevalence rates of exposure among cases and controls and the odds ratio, which is an estimate of the true relative risk. Major advantages are that it is useful to study rare diseases and diseases with long latency. The case-control-study approach is limited in that factors are "observed" after the occurrence of disease and that cases and controls are selected from two different populations.

3. *Cohort (prospective) study:* The sampling approach for this study design is based on exposure status. The incidence of disease or other health related outcome is then compared in persons exposed to the study factor and in nonexposed persons. Both groups are followed over time, that is, prospectively. It is important to note that individuals selected for the study, be they exposed or unexposed, must be free of the outcome or disease being investigated when they are first identified and selected for study. Measures of risk are *incidence (absolute risk)* and *relative risk*. The major advantage of this study design is that the study factor (exposure) level on each subject is observed at the onset of the follow-up period, before the disease or outcome is observed. The cohort study design is limited in that it is not useful for rare diseases or diseases of long latency period and it takes a long time to complete. There are two subtypes of cohort studies, the *concurrent* and the *nonconcurrent* types. These basic designs are essentially the same with the exception that the nonconcurrent type abbreviates the period of follow-up by beginning the study in the present but tracks the exposure from some point in the past. This type of nonconcurrent study is also referred to as a *historical prospective study*.

A variety of sampling procedures are employed combining elements from more than one study design; these are known as *hybrid study designs*. An example is a *nested case-control study,* which is a case-control study nested in a cohort design.

Experimental studies are studies involving manipulation of the study factor by the investigator and where randomization is used to allocate subjects to study groups. There are several types of experimental studies:

1. *Clinical trial (randomized controlled trial, or RCT):* This calls for the random assignment of individuals to treatments, preferably using a double-blind approach. This study design can be divided into *therapeutic, intervention* or *prevention trials*. It is considered to

be the most scientifically rigorous type of study or the gold standard for evaluating scientific evidence. Randomization has a number of advantages. It eliminates selection bias on the part of participants and investigators; it tends to create groups that are comparable in all factors that influence prognosis, whether these be known or unknown; and it gives validity to the statistical treatment of the data.

2. *Community intervention trial*: This is an experiment in which the allocation of treatments or preventive interventions is to communities rather than to individuals. This approach, used frequently in community-based research, is described in detail in chapter 9.

3. *Laboratory experiment*: This is an experiment of short duration and is used to estimate acute biological or behavioral responses that are believed to be risk factors for the disease under study. All three of these experimental study designs have limitations in that the study population may differ from the target population, because the sample was carefully selected to meet the criteria of the experiment. The practicality of implementing the design is the most often cited limitation; for example, randomization of patients may not be ethical.

4. *Evaluation studies*: Epidemiologic methods can be used to evaluate the effectiveness of (nonresearch) prevention and control programs. The design is similar to the cohort study, where "exposure" is defined as exposure to a health program. The use of a comparison group, or a nonexposed group that does not receive the evaluated program, allows one to determine what effect the prevention or control program had on the outcome under study. A variety of methods can be used to select and identify a comparison group, including random assignment (experimental), nonrandom assignment (quasi-experimental), and the use of a historical comparison group.

Quasi-experimental studies are studies in which the study factor has been artificially manipulated by the investigator but randomization has not been used.

A detailed discussion of epidemiologic study designs is usually found in basic textbooks of epidemiology and survey methodology. The flow chart in Figure 5.1 summarizes information on the grouping of study designs such as the experimental, observational, descriptive, and analytical studies that have been discussed (Chekoway, Pearce, & Crawford-Brown, 1989; Gordis, 1996; Kelsey, Petitti, & King, 1998; Kleinbaum, Kupper, & Morgenstern, 1986; Lilienfeld & Stolley, 1994;

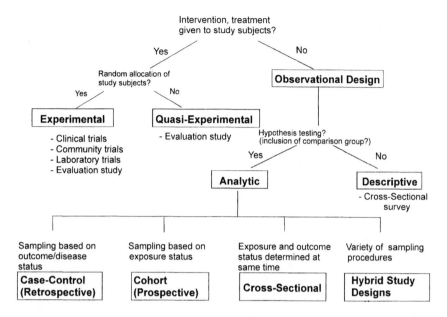

FIGURE 5.1 Identifying epidemiologic study designs.

Mausner, Kramer, & Bahn, 1985; Timmreck, 1998; Weisberg, Krosnick, & Bowen, 1996).

Table 5.1 provides a summary of the advantages and disadvantages of each of the major study designs that have been described.

DESCRIPTIVE STUDIES

Descriptive studies, also referred to as descriptive epidemiology, are concerned with the study of the distribution of disease, disability, injury, and death in population groups. Descriptive epidemiology summarizes in a systematic fashion the basic data on health and the factors related to the major causes of disease and death. The objectives of descriptive epidemiology are: (a) to evaluate trends in health and disease among populations and population subgroups; (b) to assist in the planning, provision, and evaluation of health services; (c) to identify problems to be studied by analytic epidemiologic methods; and (d) to identify nonrandom variations in the distribution of disease and generate

TABLE 5.1   Summary of Advantages and Disadvantages of Epidemiologic Study Designs

Type of Study	Advantages	Disadvantages
Cross-Sectional *Prevalence*	Provides a sort of snapshot of population. Usually based on general population (good for generalizability). Can be done quickly.	Cannot determine temporal sequence of cause and effect. People who quickly recover or die from a disease have less chance of being included in the study. Persons with disease in remission maybe falsely classified as not having the disease. Not appropriate for rare disease, or those of short duration.
Case-Control *Retrospective*	Quick and inexpensive in comparison to other designs. Appropriate for evaluating diseases with long latent periods, and for rare diseases. Multiple factors can be evaluated for a single disease.	Information on potential risk factors and confounding variables may be difficult to verify. Difficult to assess whether disease causes exposure to agent, or the exposure causes the disease. Difficult to identify and assemble case group representatives and identify appropriate control group.
Cohort *Prospective*	Lack of bias in exposure. Yields relative risk and incidence rates. Can study additional disease associations.	Very costly. Large number of subjects. Long follow-up period. Not suitable for rare diseases. Problems of attrition. Changes over time in criteria and methods.
Experimental *Clinical or Community Trials*	Rigorous methodology. Assesses efficacy of new drugs, treatments, or interventions. Random assignment minimizes confounding.	May not be feasible, or ethical, in public health practice. Study population may be different from target population.
Evaluation Studies	Studies effectiveness of programs or interventions. Can use randomized or nonrandomized designs.	Appropriate comparison group may not be available. Identification and control of confounding may be difficult.

hypotheses to be tested. Describing the occurrence of disease in the community includes an analysis of who is affected, and where and when the cases or deaths occur. Thus, descriptive epidemiology focuses on characteristics related to *person*, *place* and *time*.

Person

Among the many characteristics of a person, the most important and the ones routinely studied in epidemiology are those of age, gender, race and ethnicity, education, marital status, and occupation. Among these demographic variables, *age* is the most important. Mortality and morbidity rates of almost all conditions show some relationship to age. Age predicts differences in disease, disability, injury, and death. For example, the prevalence of arthritis increases with age (Table 5.2). Age is related not only to the risk of disease, in many cases, but also to severity. An estimated 8 million persons (3% of the U.S. population) experience activity limitation due to arthritis, with the highest rates among those aged 65 years and older (Table 5.2).

Age-specific death rates for all causes of death regardless of gender and race show a J-shaped pattern (Figure 5.2). These sharp differences in death rates by age require that we perform a correction "adjustment"

TABLE 5.2 Prevalence of Self-Reported Arthritis and Activity Limitations Due to Arthritis

Age (years)	Prevalence of arthritis		Rate of activity limitation caused by arthritis	
	Males	Females	Males	Females
≤ 24	0.8%	1.5%	0.1%	0.2%
25–34	5.5%	8.6%	0.5%	1.1%
35–44	10.5%	15.7%	1.3%	2.2%
45–54	19.4%	27.7%	2.1%	4.9%
55–64	29.7%	40.9%	5.2%	9.4%
65–74	44.5%	52.2%	7.1%	11.6%
75–84	46.4%	61.1%	8.0%	15.1%
85	42.1%	63.3%	10.3%	20.1%

Note: From Centers for Disease Control and Prevention, "Prevalence of Arthritis—United States, 1997," 2001, *Morbidity and Mortality Weekly Report, 50*(17), pp. 334–336. Adapted with permission.

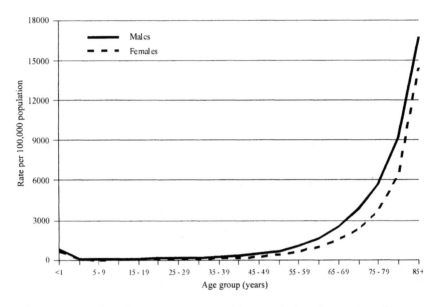

FIGURE 5.2   Death rates per 100,000 population by age and gender.

Note: From National Center for Health Statistics. (2000). *Deaths: Final Data for 1998.*

for any age differences that exist between two population groups we are comparing.

Gender is another important characteristic among the person variables. Overall, death rates are higher for males than for females. In 1998, the age-adjusted death rate for all causes of death combined was 58% higher for males than for females (Murphy, 2000). Gender differences in mortality also vary by specific diseases. In 1998, the greatest gender differential in age-adjusted mortality rates was for suicide (4.3 male deaths to one female death), followed by homicide (3.5:1) and accidents (2.4:1). For stroke and hypertension, the ratio of male to female deaths was 1.1:1, and for Alzheimer's disease the ratio was 0.9:1. Gender differences in mortality are observed within each race and ethnicity category, as well (Figure 5.3). Despite the higher mortality rate among males as compared to females, morbidity rates are generally higher in females. According to the 1999 National Ambulatory Medical Care Survey, females made 58.9% of all physician office visits, and the visit rate was higher for females than for males in the age

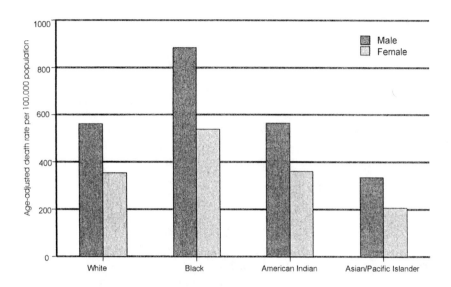

FIGURE 5.3.   Age adjusted death rates by race and gender: United States, 1998.

Note: From National Center for Health Statistics. (2000, July 17). *National Ambulatory Medical Care Survey: 1999 Summary.*

groups between 15 and 64 years (Cherry, Burt, & Woodwell, 2001). The reason women have a higher rate of illness and physician contact but less mortality may be due to a number of factors, including difference in risk associated with differences in genetics, hormonal balances, environment, or lifestyle. In addition, women seek medical care more freely and perhaps at an earlier stage of disease. Thus, the same disease will tend to have a less lethal course in women than in men.

The occurrence of death, disease, and other public health problems is often disproportionately higher in racial and ethnic minority populations as well. *Race* and *ethnicity* are important, yet controversial, components of public health surveillance and vital statistics data collection systems. Recently, the purpose and process of collecting information on race and ethnicity have been debated (Krieger et al., 1993; Oppenheimer, 2001; Thomas, 2001). Current racial categories may be too broad to be meaningful and may not allow for multiracial heritage.

Information on race and ethnicity has traditionally been used to identify differences in health status among population subgroups. Disparities in mortality and morbidity have been observed. Overall, in 1998 age-adjusted deaths rates for Blacks exceed those of Whites by 53% (Murphy, 2000). Death rates from stroke are substantially higher among Blacks as compared to Whites, for all age groups except 85+ (Figure 5.4). Infant mortality rates among Black infants remain nearly twice that for White infants. Disparities in risk behaviors also exist. Native Americans use tobacco at substantially higher rates than any other subgroup. In Oklahoma, over 30% of adults currently smoke cigarettes (Bolen, Rhodes, Powell-Griner, Bland, & Holtzman, 2000). Among Native American youth, approximately 50% report current use of cigarettes and/or smokeless tobacco (Oklahoma State Department of Health, 1999).

Differences in rates of mortality and morbidity by race may reflect more important determinants of health. Instead, race may be a marker for other underlying problems of greater relevance to health, including socioeconomic status, cultural or behavioral characteristics, environment, lifestyle, and accessibility and quality of medical care. Clearly, additional research is required to fully understand racial differences in health status.

Socioeconomic status describes an individual's position in society and is associated with health-related characteristics, as well as morbidity and mortality. Socioeconomic disparities in health are related to an

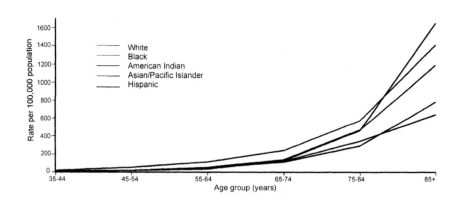

FIGURE 5.4. Death rates from stroke by age and race/ethnicity, United States, 1997.

Note: From *Morbidity and Mortality Weekly Report, 49*(05), 94–97, 2001, February 11.

individual's access to social and economic resources. A socioeconomic gradient exists for most health indicators examined, including health care access and utilization. Socioeconomic status is widely used in public health studies to identify groups at higher risk for specific diseases.

Socioeconomic status is often based on various measures, including level of education, type of occupation, household or family income, and poverty status, each of which has its own advantages and disadvantages. Income is the most common measure of socioeconomic status. It provides a direct measure of the quality of resources to which an individual has access, such as food, housing, and health care. Income, however, is often not reported on an individual basis. Converting family income into a percentage of the federal poverty level takes family size into account. Education, a frequently used measure of socioeconomic status, may be more accurately and completely reported. Although occupation reflects both education and income, it may not be relevant for some subgroups, such as children, retired persons, and women who are not currently employed.

Socioeconomic differences in risk factors, such as smoking, are common (Figure 5.5). For both men and women, the highest smoking prevalence rates are observed among those with less than a high school education. In 1995, among men, those with the lowest level of education were nearly three times as likely to smoke as the most educated.

Marital status has been consistently observed to be associated with mortality rates in both men and women. Age-adjusted death rates by marital status show the highest mortality among those never married, followed by those who are divorced or widowed. Those who were married at the time of death have the lowest mortality (Murphy, 2000). The lower mortality rates observed among married individuals may be due to psychological and physical support of the spouse, as well as selection factors that also influence marital status. Other *family variables* of importance include family size and structure, birth order, maternal age, and parental deprivation. For example, older maternal age is associated with higher rates of congenital malformations, such as Down's syndrome.

Place

An examination of the frequency of disease relative to place of occurrence is paramount to identifying the source or etiology of disease, as

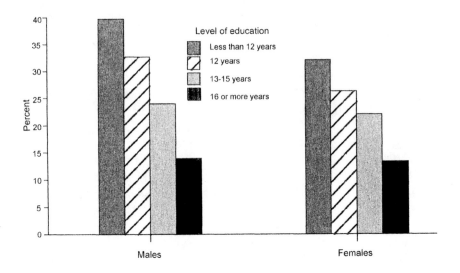

FIGURE 5.5.   Age-adjusted cigarette smoking rates among adults 25 years of age and older by education and gender: United States, 1995.

Note: From Pamuk, E., Makuc, D., Heck, K., Reuben, C., & Lochner, K. *Socioeconomic status and health chartbook. Health, United States, 1998.* Hyattsville, MD: National Center for Health Statistics. 1998.

well as the implementation of effective prevention and control measures. The outbreak of an infectious disease is identified based on the geographic location of the source of the disease as well as the reservoir of the organism. A description of morbidity and mortality in a population can be related to natural or political boundaries. Natural boundaries refer to areas set off by natural barriers, such as mountain ranges, rivers, or deserts. Natural boundaries are likely to be more useful than political boundaries in understanding the etiology of most diseases because factors such as climate and altitude, as well as the isolation of the population group inhabiting the area may provide insight into the occurrence of disease. However, political subdivisions are the most practical way of studying disease occurrence by place. Vital statistics are usually reported by administrative boundaries, such as city, county, state, country, or census tract. An examination of the frequency of disease by urban and rural status of the community provide another dimension to the association of disease with place. Underlying factors and exposure may differ significantly in urban versus rural communities. For example, crowding and pollution in urban areas may be related to the high occurrence of specific diseases, such as asthma. On the other hand, pesticides, prolonged exposure to ultraviolet light, and large mechanized equipment in rural environments are related to other forms of morbidity and mortality.

Time

The study of disease occurrence by time is a basic aspect of describing disease trends in communities. Depending on the disease or condition being described, time may be expressed in hours, weeks, months, years, or decades. Short-term diseases with short incubation periods, that is, infectious diseases, may be best related to incidence by day or week. However, chronic diseases with very long latent periods, such as most forms of cancer, are best described in terms of years or decades. The examination of morbidity and mortality data to determine time trends is best accomplished through graphs, showing the frequency of the disease by time. Three major kinds of changes with time may be identified. They are secular trends or long-term changes; cyclical changes or periodic fluctuations on an annual basis; and short-term fluctuations in disease incidence such as those described in epidemics of infectious diseases. *Secular trends* are long-term trends that take years or decades and may describe both infectious and chronic diseases. However, secular trends are most pronounced for chronic diseases, especially cancer. Figure 5.6 depicts the dramatic decline in infant mortality over the past 60 years. Such trends over time may reflect changes in incidence or survival, or may be due to artifacts such as changes in the system of reporting or diagnosing the disease. *Cyclic trends* are short-term recurrent alterations in frequency of disease. The "cycle" may be monthly, annually, or some other periodicity. Although cyclic patterns are observed in both infectious and noninfectious conditions, these trends have been most helpful in explaining trends of an infectious nature (Figure 5.7). *Time/place clustering* of disease arouses a great deal of study and interest about the possible role of common exposures or environmental conditions in their etiology.

In summary, descriptive studies provide information on the patterns of morbidity and mortality in a community according to the characteristics of person, place, and time. Routinely collected data from disease surveillance systems, vital statistics, hospital discharge records, and

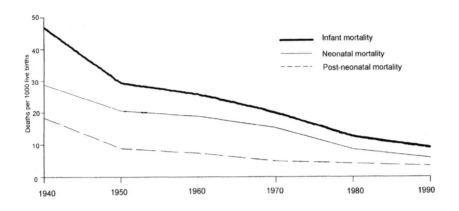

FIGURE 5.6.   Infant, neonatal, and post-neonatal mortality rates, United States, 1940–1990.

Note: From Murphy, S. L. (2000, July 24). Deaths: Final Data for 1998. *National Vital Statistics Reports, 48*(11), 87.

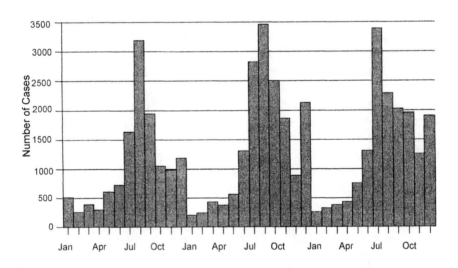

FIGURE 5.7.   Reported cases of Lyme disease by month and year, United States, 1997–1999.

Note: From *Morbidity and Mortality Weekly Report, 48*(53), 1–104, April 6, 2001; *47*(53), 1–93, Dec. 31, 1999; *46*(54), 1–87, November 20, 1998.

health surveys usually provide this information. These studies describe the distribution of disease by these variables, without regard to causal or other hypotheses (Last, 1995). Descriptive studies are hypothesis-generating; they identify health problems in the community to be studied by analytic methods.

Community health surveys and the process of identifying community assets and needs utilize the methods of descriptive epidemiology. The identification of a problem in a community and its description according to person, place, and time variables allow for a better understanding of issues related to health. In addition, this process provides valuable evidence of needs and enhances the ability to prioritize and target valuable public health and community resources

CROSS-SECTIONAL STUDIES

General Features

Cross-sectional studies are used to provide a snapshot of a population at a point in time or a period of time. Exposure status and disease (outcome) status are measured at one point in time or over a short period of time in study subjects. Figure 5.8 is a sample of a design of a

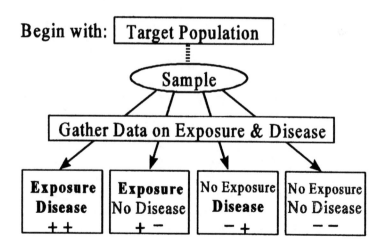

FIGURE 5.8 Design of a cross-sectional study.

cross-sectional study. Prevalence rates among those with the exposure and outcome of interest are determined; also prevalence rates of the outcome among the exposed and nonexposed are determined and compared. Because cross-sectional studies measure the extent of existing disease or exposure they are also called prevalence studies. They are most often used to learn about risk factors for diseases of slow onset and long duration for which medical care is often not sought until the disease has progressed to a relatively advanced stage.

Cross-sectional studies may be limited to assessing only the distribution of the prevalence of the exposure in the general population or to provide the measure of the burden of disease or outcome in the population. These studies are often based on a sample of the general population and must be generalized to the rest of the population.

Let us suppose we are interested in the study of the relationship between obesity (the exposure) and diabetes mellitus (the outcome) in a specified community. We then take a random or representative sample of the population in the community, and for each subject that is selected we take height and weight measurements to calculate a body mass index (BMI) (weight in kilograms divided by the square of height in meters) and use it to classify the subject(s) into weight categories such as underweight, normal weight, overweight, and obese. We then determine the presence or absence of diabetes from the subject, either by taking a history or by taking a sample of blood or urine to measure the amount of sugar and use the information to classify the subject(s) into diabetic or nondiabetic. Because we assessed the exposure (obesity) and outcome (diabetes) at the same time for each subject, we refer to this study as a cross-sectional study. Not everyone in the sample is likely to meet the criteria of either obesity, diabetes, or both. In fact, the majority of the subjects will not meet the criteria for either obesity or diabetes, but a small proportion of subjects will meet the criteria. However, those meeting the criteria of either obesity or diabetes will be counted as existing or prevalent cases of obesity and/ or diabetes. Using the illustration provided in Figure 5.8, note that in a cross-sectional study there are four groups of subjects: group 1 includes those subjects who have the exposure (obese) and the disease (diabetes); group 2 includes those subjects who have the exposure (obese) but not the disease; group 3 includes those subjects who have the disease (diabetes) but not the exposure; and group 4 includes those subjects who have neither the exposure nor the disease.

The first step in the analysis will be to calculate the number of existing (prevalent) cases with the disease (diabetes) and divide by the total number of study subjects in the sample. This will give us the prevalence rate of diabetes in the sample and therefore in the community; because the sample was a representative sample, the information obtained is generalizable. The second step will be to calculate the prevalence rate of obesity in the sample and the community by identifying the total number of subjects meeting the criteria of obesity and dividing by the total number in the study sample. It will also be useful to determine the prevalence of diabetes among the obese and the non-obese as a first step in determining whether a relationship exists between obesity and diabetes. This of course will necessitate that we display the data in what is known as a 2 × 2 table as illustrated in Table 5.3.

Selection of Study Population. The groups to be compared are sometimes selected on the basis of a characteristic or variable, particularly if the characteristics can be readily identified. For example, the exposure of interest might be membership in a certain racial or ethnic group or living in a defined geographic area. If relatively small numbers are involved, the entire population can be included. If not, then a sample can be taken. Exposure and outcome status are not measured until the sample is taken. In this case, sampling procedures must be employed to ensure sufficient representation, while maintaining an efficient study design.

Assessment of Exposure. Techniques to measure exposure status or the presence of risk factors are similar to those used in other observational study designs. Generally, questionnaires, medical or physician records, laboratory tests, physical measurements, and other special

TABLE 5.3 Illustration of Subject Selection in a Cross-Sectional Study

Exposure Status	Disease Status		
	Yes	No	TOTAL
Yes	A	B	A + B
No	C	D	C + D
TOTAL	A + C	B + D	N

procedures can be used. Date of onset and duration of exposure must also be determined to relate the exposure to the time of onset of disease. This allows assessment of dose-response relationship, a necessary ingredient for cause-effect determinations.

Measurement of Disease.   Disease status is usually determined by questionnaire, physical exam, or other special procedures. Time of onset of symptoms should be determined if possible. Diagnostic criteria should be established in advance. Criteria may be used to divide cases into definite, probable, and possible disease categories.

Advantages of Cross-sectional Studies.   As described in Table 5.1 the major advantage of this study design is that it is often based on a sample of the general population; thus, its generalizability may be considered a strength. These studies tend to be carried out over a relatively short time period, thus reducing costs. They can also be repeated in the same community.

Limitations of Cross-sectional Studies.   The temporal sequence of cause and effect relationships often cannot be determined in a cross-sectional study. A series of prevalent cases will have a higher proportion of cases with disease of long duration than a series of incident cases. People who either recover or die from a disease quickly have less chance of being included in the disease group. For some diseases, a person who is experiencing remission may be misclassified as not having the disease. Also the question of how to handle treated cases must be addressed and depends on the purpose of the study. Cross-sectional studies are not appropriate for studying rare diseases or diseases with short duration.

Basic steps in the analysis of data from cross-sectional studies can be shown from the illustration presented in Table 5.3 as follows. Prevalence of disease in exposed (A/A + B) and nonexposed (C/C + D) is first determined and then compared. Likewise, the prevalence of exposure in diseased (A/A + C) and nondiseased (B/B + D) is determined and compared in the two groups. It should be noted that the unit of observation and analysis is the individual subject. Two additional measures can be obtained from the total sample, the prevalence of the disease in the sample (A + C/N) and the prevalence of exposure in the sample (A + B/N).

Table 5.4 amplifies on the information obtained from the sample and displayed in a 2 × 2 table format. As can be seen cell A contains individual subjects who have both the exposure (obesity) and outcome of interest (diabetes) while cell B includes individuals who have only the exposure of interest (obesity) but not the disease. Cell C includes individuals with the disease (diabetes) but no exposure and cell D includes individuals with neither exposure or disease.

Example of a Cross-Sectional Study

A private drinking water and on-site sewage survey was conducted in 1996 in a rural county in Missouri (Missouri Department of Health, 1996). Geographic information software was used to take a random sample of 64 sites (wells serving individual households). Of the 64 sites, 60 were actually sampled (2 sites were served by a rural water district and 2 sites refused to participate). Water samples from wells were tested for coliform bacteria and a questionnaire was administered to residents of each household to determine gastrointestinal illness within the preceding 2 weeks. Although 197 people are represented

TABLE 5.4 Illustration of Subject Selection in a Cross-Sectional Study

Exposure Status (Obesity)	Disease Status (Diabetes)		
	Yes	No	TOTAL
Yes	Exposure (Obesity) Disease (Diabetes) ++	Exposure (Obesity) No disease + -	A + B Exposure Obesity
No	No exposure Disease (Diabetes) - +	No exposure No disease - -	C + D
TOTAL	A + C Disease (Diabetes)	B + D	N

in this survey, the unit of observation is the well. The data in Table 5.5 represent any gastrointestinal illness (GI) in the household served by the well, not the number of people reporting illness. Table 5.6 contains calculations and interpretations of the risk assessment measures in this cross-sectional study. Cases identified in a cross-sectional study are prevalent (existing) cases, rather than incident cases. When random sampling methods are used, prevalence rates can be calculated. Exposure in this example is coliform bacteria in the well water and the outcome of interest is any gastrointestinal illness among household members within the previous 2 weeks.

Ecological Studies

In an ecological study, the unit of analysis is some aggregate of individuals. An aggregate may be defined based on geographic area or as a time period. A summary measure of the frequency of exposure and a summary measure of the frequency of disease are obtained within each aggregate. For instance, data is obtained on the prevalence of smoking (per capita) for a given geographic area(s) over time and also on the age-adjusted death rates from lung cancer for the same area(s) over time. An attempt is then made to find an association between cigarette smoking and death from lung cancer by geographic areas or over a period of time in each of the geographic areas, using the aggregate data on per capita consumption of cigarettes and death rates from lung cancer. The primary feature of this "incomplete" design is that the joint distribution of the factor (smoking) and the disease (lung cancer) within the group is unknown. There are two main types of ecological studies: *The ecological comparison study*, which compares the frequency of a factor and disease in different groups. For example, one

TABLE 5.5   Example of a Cross-Sectional Study

| COLIFORM BACTERIA IN WATER | ANY GI ILLNESS IN HOUSEHOLD | | |
	Yes	No	TOTAL
Yes	8	12	20
No	6	34	40
TOTAL	14	46	60

TABLE 5.6 Description, Calculation, and Interpretation of Measures and Measures of Association

Measure	Description	Calculation	Interpretation
Proportion	Proportion exposed among diseased	8/14 = 0.571	*57.1% of households with illness had well water contaminated with coliform bacteria.*
	Proportion exposed among nondiseased	12/46 = 0.261	*26.1% of households without illness had well water contaminated with coliform bacteria.*
	Overall proportion exposed in population	20/60 = 0.333	*33.3% of study households had well water contaminated with coliform bacteria.*
Rate (risk)	Prevalence rate of disease among exposed	8/20 = 0.400	*40.0% of households with contaminated water had someone with GI illness.*
	Prevalence rate of disease among nonexposed	6/40 = 0.150	*15.0% of households without contaminated water had someone with GI illness.*
	Overall prevalence rate of disease in population	4/60 = 0.233	*23.3% of study households had someone with GI illness.*
Measures of Association	Relative risk (RR)		Can't estimate incidence rates, so can't estimate RR in cross-sectional study.
	Odds ratio (OR)	$\dfrac{8 \times 34}{12 \times 6} = 3.78$ 95% C.I., 0.93–15.9	*The odds of GI illness are 3.78 times greater in households with water contaminated by coliform bacteria than in those not contaminated.*
Attributable Risk	Attributable risk (AR) Percentage (AR%) Population attributable risk (PAR) Percentage (PAR%)		In cross-sectional studies, generally not used because incidence rates cannot be calculated.

could perform ecologic (geographic) correlations of smoking and lung cancer mortality or per capita dietary fat intake and breast cancer mortality; and *the ecological trend study*, which compares changes in frequency of exposure and disease in populations over time. For example, one could examine trends in per capita cigarette consumption in a geographic area and lung cancer death rates over a period of time, 1960–2000.

The "ecological fallacy" is an error in inference due to the failure of the study to differentiate between correlation of a factor and disease within a *population* versus within *individuals*.

Because information on the prevalence of risk factors and diseases in the population is needed on a continuous basis to examine trends over time and evaluate the impact of public health policies or intervention programs, a number of national morbidity surveys, using a cross-sectional study design, have been conducted in the United States population. The National Health Survey, begun in 1960, continues to provide information about the prevalence of morbid conditions and risk factors in the general population of the United States (Jekel, 1984; National Center for Health Statistics [NCHS], 1963). Several survey activities are included in the National Health Survey; they include the National Health Interview Survey (NHIS), the National Health and Nutrition Examination Survey (NHANES), and the National Health Record Survey (NHRS). Findings from these surveys are published by the National Center for Health Statistics in color-coded booklets known as the Rainbow Series (Jekel, 1984).

The National Health Interview Survey is a continuous, nationwide, in-person survey based on personal interviews of a sample of about 40,000 U.S. households. It has been conducted by the U.S. Census Bureau for the National Center for Health Statistics since 1957. Each week, a sample of households is interviewed and the findings are combined to provide estimates of illness in the U.S. Doctor visits and hospital stays, acute and chronic conditions, health status indicators, and limitation of activities are obtained. Additional supplemental sets of questions are asked from time to time regarding smoking habits, knowledge and attitude about major public health problems such as HIV/AIDS, and health promotion practices (Chyba & Washington, 1990; Jekel, 1984; NCHS, 1998).

The National Health and Nutrition Examination Survey (NHANES), begun in 1971, is carried out over a period of 5 to 7 years for selected age groups (NHANES I, 1971–1975, 1–74 years of age; NHANES II,

1976–1980, 6 months–74 years of age; NHANES III, 1988–1994, 2 months and up with oversampling of Blacks and Mexican Americans). It is designed to assess the health and nutrition status of adults and children through interviews and direct physical examination. The examination components consist of dental and medical examinations, laboratory tests, and psychological and physiological measurements for selected diseases. The data are used to estimate the prevalence of risk factors, major diseases and nutritional disorders. Beginning in 1999, NHANES has been carried out continuously (NCHS, 1999). In order to assess the health status of the Hispanic population of the U.S., a special Hispanic Health and Nutrition Examination Survey (HHANES) was conducted from 1982 to 1984 (Kovar, 1989).

The Health Record Survey provides information on samples of institutions and facilities providing medical care and health services (Jekel, 1984; Kovar, 1989). Since 1965, information about discharge diagnoses of a sample of patients admitted to short-stay hospitals is provided by the National Hospital Discharge Survey. The National Ambulatory Medical Care Survey, conducted annually from 1974 to 1981 and then once every 4 years beginning in 1985, provides information on patient complaints and the diagnoses made by physicians in private offices.

The Behavioral Risk Factor Surveillance System (BRFSS) and the Youth Risk Behavior Surveillance System (YRBSS) have become very important sources of prevalent data on a number of lifestyle factors and screening practices for major diseases among adults and youth in the United States. The BRFSS is an ongoing system of surveys conducted by the Centers for Disease Control and Prevention and state health departments. It is a cross-sectional telephone survey on noninstitutionalized adults who are 18 years of age and older. The BRFSS uses a multistage cluster design based on random digit dialing technique that attempts to identify a random sample from each state's residents. State data are pooled to provide nationally representative estimates (Nelson, Holtzman, Waller, Leutzinger, & Condon, 1998; Waksberg, 1978). Because the methods are consistent from state to state and year to year, the information is comparable between and among states and with national data. Data obtained through telephone interviews is limited to those households with telephones, and therefore the estimates obtained are generalizable only to those with telephones. It is estimated that about 5% of U.S. households do not have telephones, but the estimates vary by state and racial or ethnic group.

The YRBSS consists of a representative sample of 9th- through 12th-grade high school students from the 50 states and the District of

Columbia. It consists of a biennial, nationwide, state, and local school-based survey using a self-administered questionnaire.Direct comparison of data from this survey should be done with caution as a variety of sampling methods have been used and the quality of the data varies from state to state (Centers for Disease Control and Prevention [CDC], 1995, 1996, 1998).

In summary, cross-sectional studies are used to assess the prevalence of health-related states at one point in time or a period of time by selecting a sample of the population without regard to either the outcome or exposure. They can be either descriptive or analytical in nature depending on the objectives of the study. The major strength of cross-sectional studies is their generalizability when proper sampling methods are utilized. They are also cost-effective. The National Health Surveys conducted by the National Center for Health Statistics and the Behavioral Risk Factor Surveillance System carried out by the Centers for Disease Control and Prevention and state departments of health are examples of well-known cross-sectional studies.

SAMPLING ISSUES IN CROSS-SECTIONAL STUDIES

Use of Sampling to Determine Disease Prevalence in the Community

As mentioned earlier, cross-sectional studies can be either descriptive—that is, provide quantitative estimates of the magnitude of a health problem in the population, be it an exposure variable or a disease outcome—or analytical, that is, used to test a hypothesis on the relationship between a given exposure and the outcome of interest. They can also be used to obtain information on the knowledge, attitudes, beliefs, behaviors, and practices of a large or small segment of the population or community. There are two types of approaches that can be used to assess the magnitude of the public health problem being investigated in the population and people's knowledge, attitudes, beliefs, behaviors, and practices. One is to collect information on every subject in the population or community, which can be prohibitively expensive, or to carefully select a sample of the population and then use the information to draw inference to the rest of the population or community. The size of the community, available resources, and time usually dictate the approach taken by the investigator. Given the large size of communities being studied, such as counties, states, or nations, and the cost involved in studying these communities, the most common approach used in cross-sectional studies is selecting a sample of the population. There are two main categories of sampling, defined according to how the sample was selected: *probability samples* and *nonprobability samples*. A probability sample has the feature that every element in the population has a known nonzero chance of being included in the sample. Nonprobability samples do not have this feature. Nonprobability or convenient samples, when used, are not representative of the population or community being studied (Barnett, 1991; Levy & Lemeshaw, 1991; Weisberg et al., 1996).

Probability samples include random (simple) samples, systematic samples, stratified samples, cluster samples, and multistage samples. It is important to use scientifically sound sampling methods when conducting cross-sectional studies. The basic purpose of sampling is to save money and time. Sampling may result in greater accuracy (Barnett, 1991; Levy & Lemeshow, 1991; Weisberg et al., 1996).

Sampling Methods

Random sample, commonly known as *simple random sample*, is defined as a sample that is selected in such a way that every possible element or unit in the population has a fixed and determined probability or chance of being selected, that is, has an equal and independent chance of being selected. Random samples require counting of all potential subjects before sampling begins, an extensive process that may not always be feasible to implement. This is carried out by assigning a number from 1 to N. Numbers are then selected at random from a table of random numbers until the desired sample size is attained. The two major advantages of random sampling from a population are (a) the chances of bias are minimized or eliminated, and (b) probability statements may be employed in the evaluation of results, that is, it enables the investigator to determine the reliability of the results. For a random sample, the only source of sampling error is random variation resulting from the size of the sample and the heterogeneity of the population being studied. If a sample is selected in such a way that gives each member of the population an equal chance of being selected, then it is a random sample (Barnett, 1991; Last, 1995; Levy & Lemeshaw, 1991; Weisberg et al., 1996).

Systematic sample is defined in such a way that the unit sampled or study subjects are selected according to some simple, systematic rule, such as equal interval, choosing every *n*th individual from a list of subjects, selecting all persons whose names begin with specified alphabetic letters, choosing those born on a certain date, or those located at specified points on a master list. Sometimes systematic samples are more representative than simple random samples. However, the potential for bias is increased when selection is based on names beginning with a specified alphabetic letters, knowing that some names for certain ethnic groups are more likely to use certain letters of the alphabet than others. Because it is possible to perform systematic sampling at the same time that a sampling frame is being assembled, systematic sampling is the most widely used sampling approach (Barnett, 1991; Last, 1995; Levy & Lemeshaw, 1991; Weisberg et al., 1996).

Stratified sample, also known as *stratified random sample*, is defined as a sample in which the population is divided or partitioned into several distinct strata or subgroups such as age, gender, race, or socioeconomic status, then a random sample is selected from each of the strata or subgroups according to the size of the population in each. It is important that the population be divided into mutually exclusive and exhaustive strata. For instance if the subgroups are divided equally into five major age groups and each age group has 20% of the total population, then the random samples of each of the strata will provide an equal number of samples representing 20% of the total sample selected. The more homogeneous the strata are, the more precise the estimates will be. It is appropriate to refer to it as a stratified random sample when simple random sampling is used within each stratum (Barnett, 1991; Last, 1995; Levy & Lemeshaw, 1991; Weisberg et al., 1996).

Cluster sampling is a sampling method in which the sampling unit or cluster includes a group of persons rather than an individual. The cluster may be a city block, a county, a school, or a file drawer. The listing unit in such clusters may be the household, hospital, classroom, or individual file folder. Further, the elementary unit in each of the listing units of the clusters may be a person, patient, students, or account. (Barnett, 1991; Last, 1995; Levy & Lemeshaw, 1991; Weisberg et al., 1996). It should be noted that different statistical procedures are required for different sampling methods.

Nonprobability samples, also known as *quota samples, haphazard samples, volunteer samples,* and *purposive or judgmental samples,* are frequently used in public opinion surveys or market research. They are used to get around the expense, feasibility, and time issues associated with probability sampling. For instance, in a *quota survey* the interviewer is asked to contact and interview five individuals from each of six racial/gender subgroups. It is left up to the interviewer to decide how these individuals are selected. It is possible that the interviewer may decide to select all the racial/gender groups from one geographic area known for its affluence and also for its convenience, thus meeting the quota by selecting a sample that is not representative of the racial group in the whole population. The main advantage of a quota sample is the willingness of the respondents to participate, while its main drawback is its sources of bias, such as its tendency to include the middle class disproportionately. In *purposive* or *judgmental sampling*, individuals are selected because they are considered to be the most representative of the population as a whole (Barnett, 1991; Levy & Lemeshaw, 1991; Weisberg et al., 1996). For instance, an opinion survey is conducted at a grocery store to assess the customers' preference for certain food items being introduced. Certain busy days (for instance, Saturdays) are selected to conduct the survey to avoid unusual days when the customer traffic may be slow. This may lead to more valid and reliable estimates than the approach of using a random sample of days. Purposive sampling reduces the potential for including atypical days. The main advantages of a purposive sample are its low cost and the fact that it uses the best available information. One disadvantage is the potential for including unknown sources of bias. The main advantage of a haphazard or convenient sample is the availability of the sample; the main disadvantage is that there is no necessary relationship to the population being sampled. Likewise, volunteer samples are used because they ensure the cooperation of the subjects who are being asked to participate, but the main drawback is that they are not representative of the population. Table 5.7 summarizes the advantages and disadvantages of all types of probability and nonprobability samples.

SUMMARY

There are two main types of sampling used, probability and nonprobability sampling. Nonprobability sampling, such as quota samples, haphazard samples, volunteer samples, and purposive or judgmental samples are used in market research and public opinion surveys. They are primarily selected because of convenience, low cost, and accessi-

TABLE 5.7　Advantages and Disadvantages of Probability and Nonprobability Samples

Types of Samples

Sampling Method	Advantages	Disadvantages
Nonprobability		
Purposive sample	Inexpensive Uses best available information	No estimates of accuracy May miss important elements
Volunteer subjects	Cooperative respondents	Not representative of population
Haphazard sample	Available sample	No necessary relation to population
Quota sample	Willing respondents	Middle-class and other biases
Probability		
Simple random sample	Accuracy can be estimated Sampling error can be estimated	Expensive interviews too dispersed and full list required
Systematic selection procedure	Convenience	Periodicity in list
Stratified sample	Guarantees adequate representation of groups Usually decreased error	Sometimes requires weighting
Cluster sample	Decreased cost	Increased error
Multistage area sample	Lower cost than simple random sample for large populations Lower error than cluster	Higher error than simple random sample Higher cost than cluster

Note: From Weisberg, Krosnick, & Bowen, 1996.

bility, but are limited because of lack of representation, generalizability, and accuracy. Probability samples such as simple random, systematic, stratified, cluster, and multistage samples are most commonly used in cross-sectional surveys to assess health and disease conditions in the population. When properly done, they can provide an accurate assessment of the prevalence of the health-related states and conditions in the population being surveyed. Because they are representative samples, generalizability is assured.

REFERENCES

Barnett, V. (1991). *Sample survey: Principles & methods.* New York: Oxford University Press.

Bolen, J. C., Rhodes, L., Powell-Griner, E. E., Bland, S. D., & Holtzman, D. (2000). *State-specific prevalence of selected health behaviors by race and ethnicity— behavioral risk factor surveillance system, 1997.*

Centers for Disease Control and Prevention. (1995). Youth risk behavior surveillance—United States, 1993. *Morbidity and Mortality Weekly Report, 45*(SS-4).

Centers for Disease Control and Prevention. (1996). Youth risk behavior surveillance—United States, 1995. *Morbidity and Mortality Weekly Report, 45*(SS-4).

Centers for Disease Control and Prevention. (1998). Youth risk behavior surveillance—United States, 1997. *Morbidity and Mortality Weekly Report, 47*(SS-3).

Checkoway, H., Pearce, N. E., & Crawford-Brown, D. J. (1989). *Research methods in occupational epidemiology.* New York: Oxford University Press.

Cherry, D. K., Burt, C. W., & Woodwell, D. A. (2001). *National Ambulatory Medical Care Survey: 1999 Summary. Advance data from vital and health statistics* (No. 322). Hyattsville, MD: National Center for Health Statistics.

Chyba, M. M., & Washington, L. R. (1990). Questionnaires from the National Health Interview Survey, 1980–84. National Center for Health Statistics. *Vital Health Statistics, 1, 24.*

Flanders, W. D., Lin, L., Pirkle, J. L., & Caudill, S. P. (1992). Assessing the direction of causality in cross-sectional studies. *American Journal of Epidemiology, 135,* 926–935.

Friis, R. H., & Sellers, T. A. (1999). *Epidemiology for public health practice* (2nd ed.). Gaithersburg, MD: Aspen.

Gordis, L. (1996). *Epidemiology.* Philadelphia: W. B. Saunders.

Jekel, J. F. (1984). The rainbow reviews: Publications of the National Center for Health Statistics. *Journal of Chronic Disease, 37,* 681–688.

Jekel, J. F., Elmore, J. G., & Katz, D. L. (1996). *Epidemiology, biostatistics and preventive medicine.* Philadelphia: W. B. Saunders.

Kelsey, J. L., Petitti, D. B., & King, A. C. (1998). Key methodologic concepts and issues. In R. C. Brownson & D. B. Petitti (Eds.), *Applied epidemiology: Theory to practice.* New York: Oxford University Press.

Kelsey, J. L., Whittemore, A. S., Evans, A. S., & Thompson, W. D. (1998). *Methods in observational epidemiology* (2nd ed.). New York: Oxford University Press.

Kleinbaum, D. G., Kupper, L. L., & Morgenstern, H. M. (1986). *Epidemiologic research.* Belmont, CA: Lifetime Learning.

Kovar, M. G. (1989). Data systems of the National Center for Health Statistics. National Center for Health Statistics. *Vital Health Statistics, 1,* 23.

Krieger, N., Rowley, D., Herman, A. A., et al. (1993). Racism, sexism, and social class: Implications for studies of health disease and well-being. *American Journal of Preventive Medicine, 9,* 82–122.

Last, J. M. (Eds.). (1995). *A dictionary of epidemiology* (3rd ed.). New York: Oxford University Press.

Levy, P. S., & Lemeshow, S. (1991). *Sampling of populations: Methods and applications.* New York: Wiley.

Lilienfeld, D. E., & Stolley, P. D. (1994). *Foundations of epidemiology* (3rd ed.). New York: Oxford University Press.

Mausner, J. S., Kramer, S., & Bahn, A. (1985). *Epidemiology—An introductory text.* Philadelphia: W. B. Saunders.

Murphy, S. L. (2000). Deaths: Final data for 1998. (1996, July 24). *National Vital Statistics Reports, 48*(11), 1–106.

Missouri Department of Health. (1996). Unpublished data.

National Center for Health Statistics. (1963). *Origin, program, and operation of the U.S. National Health Survey.* PHS Publication No.100, Series 1, No. 1. U.S. Department of Health, Education, and Welfare. Washington, DC: U.S. Government Printing Office.

National Center for Health Statistics. (1998). *Data file documentation, National Health Interview Survey, 1995* [machine readable data file and documentation, CD-ROM Series 10. 10C]. Hyattsville, MD: National Center for Health Statistics.

National Center for Health Statistics. (1999). National Center for Health Statistics Programs and Activities. Hyattsville, MD: Centers for Disease Control and Prevention, U.S. Department of Health and Human Services.

Nelson, D. E., Holtzman, D., Waller, M., Leutzinger, C. L., & Condon, K. (1998, August 10). Objectives and design of the Behavioral Risk Factor Surveillance System. *Proceedings of the Section on Survey Methods of the American Statistical Association National Meeting,* Dallas, TX.

Oklahoma State Department of Health. (1999). *Oklahoma Youth Tobacco Survey.* 1999: Summary Report. Oklahoma City, OK: Office of Tobacco Use Prevention.

Oppenheimer, G. M. (2001, July). Paradigm lost: Race, ethnicity and the search for a new population taxonomy. *American Journal of Public Health, 91*(7), 1049–1055.

Pamuk, E., Makuc, D., Heck, K., Reuben, C., & Lochner, K. (1998). *Socioeconomic status and health chartbook. Health, United States, 1998.* Hyattsville, MD: National Center for Health Statistics.

Thomas, S. B. (2001, July). The color line: Race matters in the elimination of health disparities. *American Journal of Public Health, 91*(7), 1046–1048.

Timmreck, T. C. (1998). *An introduction to epidemiology* (2nd ed.). Boston: Jones & Bartlett.

Waksberg, J. S. (1978). Methods for random digit dialing. *Journal of the American Statistical Association, 73*, 40–46.

Weisberg, H. F., Krosnick, J. A., & Bowen, B. D. (1996). *An introduction to survey research, polling, and data analysis* (3rd ed.). Thousand Oaks, CA: Sage.

Chapter 6

THE BEHAVIORAL RISK FACTOR SURVEILLANCE SYSTEM

Deborah Holtzman

The U.S. Behavioral Risk Factor Surveillance System (BRFSS), a state-based system of telephone health surveys, was established in 1984 by the Centers for Disease Control and Prevention (CDC) (Frazier, Franks, & Anderson, 1992; Holtzman, Powell-Griner, Bolen, & Rhodes, 2000). Information on health risk behaviors, clinical preventive health practices, and selected health conditions, primarily related to chronic disease and injury, is obtained from a representative sample of adults in each state. Data are collected monthly in all 50 states, the District of Columbia, Puerto Rico, and most recently, Guam; annual point-in-time surveys are conducted in the Virgin Islands. Currently, close to 200,000 adult interviews are completed each year, making the BRFSS the largest telephone health survey in the world.

The BRFSS has a relatively long history in behavioral surveillance (McQueen, 1996). A number of events came together in the United States that culminated in the development of the system in the early 1980s. One important factor was a greater awareness of the impact of personal or lifestyle behaviors (e.g., smoking, lack of exercise) on chronic illness and disease (Anderson et al., 1988). At the time, however, there was little empirical evidence (at least from the general population) to support these associations. Some data were available from periodic surveys at the national level, but these data were not necessarily relevant for states that needed information on which to base their individual health-promotion efforts. About the same time, the telephone emerged as a reliable and affordable alternative to other types of data collection methods, notably in-person household surveys (Groves & Kahn, 1979).

As a result, CDC developed a system that could be administered at the state level, whereby data could be collected over the telephone from a sample of adults residing in each state. The basic philosophy was to collect data on actual behaviors rather than attitudes or knowledge, and to focus on chronic rather than communicable diseases. Such behavioral data were thought to be especially useful for planning, implementing, monitoring, and evaluating health promotion and disease prevention programs to reduce morbidity and mortality.

To determine the feasibility of behavioral surveillance, initial point-in-time state surveys were conducted in 29 states from 1981 to 1983 (Gentry et al., 1985; Marks et al., 1985). In 1984, the BRFSS was established by CDC, with 15 states participating in monthly data collection. A standard core questionnaire was developed by CDC to provide data that could be compared across states. Except for physical activity, for which there were no standard questions available, the survey included existing questions from national surveys such as the National Health Interview Survey (NHIS) and National Heart, Lung, and Blood Institute surveys on hypertension. Data were collected on the six individual-level risk factors associated with the leading causes of premature mortality among adults: cigarette smoking, alcohol use, physical inactivity, diet, hypertension, and safety belt use. The initial questionnaire was designed to last no more than 10 minutes so that states could add questions of their own choosing.

THE FEDERAL-STATE PARTNERSHIP

Although designed as a cooperative federal-state venture, most decisions about the BRFSS during the first several years were made by staff at CDC. This occurred primarily because of limited state capacity in the areas of survey methodology, questionnaire development, and data analysis. Consequently, the questionnaire was designed by CDC staff with informal input from interested state personnel. For the remainder of the 1980s, most modifications to the basic questionnaire were made by individuals or groups at CDC with interest and expertise in certain subject areas.

As new states entered the system and participating states became increasingly involved in survey operations, development of the questionnaire became a more cooperative federal-state activity in 1990. At the same time, this partnership was formalized with the creation of the BRFSS Working Group. The group, which is comprised of selected BRFSS state representatives and CDC staff, meets regularly during the year. States are now actively involved in all discussions concerning proposed changes to the questionnaire. Moreover, since 1998, all new or substantially revised questions must undergo cognitive testing. However, final decision-making authority for questionnaire content and wording continues to rest with CDC.

Using computer-assisted telephone interviewing (CATI) techniques, participating states are responsible for collecting data each month from a representative sample of adult residents in their states. For data collection, CDC initially encouraged states to use cluster designs based on the Waksberg method (Waksberg, 1978); however, even for the initial 29 point-in-time surveys, there was state variability; nine of these states used simple random samples. Because data collection was a state activity, some variability in sampling methodology continued. Over time, an increasing number of states moved to disproportionate stratified sampling (DSS), which was viewed as more cost-effective.

Because the BRFSS was established as a federal-state partnership, responsibilities are specified through a cooperative agreement that details the role of each partner. At the state level, all BRFSS activities are situated in the state health department. The state program oversees all aspects of data collection, including hiring appropriate staff, ensuring that interviews are conducted according to protocol, and training and evaluating interviewers. Other duties include data editing, forwarding the data to CDC for processing, and working to achieve CDC quality assurance goals. States also are involved in analysis and reporting of the data.

At CDC, responsibility for the BRFSS lies with the Behavioral Surveillance Branch which is located in the Division of Adult and Community Health in the National Center for Chronic Disease Prevention and Health Promotion. The Behavioral Surveillance Branch is responsible for purchasing randomly generated telephone-number samples, programming the states' questionnaires for CATI, editing monthly data files, reformatting data to adhere to a common CDC standard, generating quality control reports to facilitate monitoring activities, and computing annual weighting factors. It is also responsible for producing data sets for analysis; preparing annual tabular summaries of BRFSS data for each state, including cross-tabulations by demographic variables;

and preparing annual summary prevalence reports reflecting estimates across states for selected variables. In addition, the branch collaborates and provides assistance to states for data collection, analysis, interpretation, and utilization, and coordinates and facilitates the exchange of technical information among states.

CHANGES IN THE DESIGN OF THE BRFSS QUESTIONNAIRE

Because of the ability to obtain representative state-level data and the absence of comparable data collection systems, the BRFSS was recognized by the late 1980s as a unique mechanism for obtaining health data. As a result, other programs both at CDC and in state health departments became interested in using the BRFSS. Gradually, the size of the questionnaire increased as new subject areas were added.

Selection of new subject areas for the BRFSS is based on input from states and CDC about priority topics, as well as additional financial support, primarily at the federal level. The BRFSS core questionnaire now contains questions on HIV/AIDS, health care access, cancer screening and other clinical preventive services, and additional tobacco-related questions. This greater interest and support allowed expansion of the BRFSS to 50 states by 1993 (participation in the 1993 BRFSS included the District of Columbia and all states except Wyoming), and to gradually increase the overall number of completed interviews to an average of almost 2,300 per state by 1995.

In addition to changes to the core questionnaire, CDC-supported modules (one or more questions on a single topic, e.g., smokeless tobacco, quality of life) were offered to states beginning in 1988. These modules have almost always been the result of other CDC centers or divisions within the National Center for Chronic Disease Prevention and Health Promotion proposing sets of questions on subjects of interest. More recently, other federal programs outside of CDC have submitted proposals to add questions (e.g., Health Services Research Administration, Administration on Aging, Veterans Administration). This activity has grown substantially, and in 2000, 19 modules were supported from which states could select.

Over the years, there was general agreement among states and CDC that the BRFSS core questionnaire would not exceed 80 questions

so that states could continue to include their own questions and selected optional modules. By the early 1990s, there was no room for
additional expansion of the BRFSS core. To address this situation, a
long-term plan was proposed by the BRFSS Working Group in 1992
(Table 6.1). Under this plan, a rotating core was established, whereby
questions on certain topics would be asked every other year, for example, nutrition and physical activity in even-numbered years; injury
control, alcohol, cholesterol screening, and hypertension in odd-num-
bered years.

A second part of the 1992 BRFSS long term plan was to include up
to five emerging core questions to the questionnaire. This option was
added primarily to test questions in new subject areas; if these questions were found to be useful, they could eventually be added either
to the core questionnaire or to a CDC-supported module. Emerging

TABLE 6.1. The BRFSS Questionnaire Long-Term Plan, 1993–2000

Fixed Core		Rotating Core I (odd years)		Rotating Core II (even years)	
Topic	Number of questions	Topic	Number of questions	Topic	Number of questions
Health status	4	Hyperten-sion	3	Physical activity	10
Health insurance	3	Injury	5	Fruits & vegetables	6
Routine check-up	1	Alcohol	5	Weight control	6
Diabetes	1	Immuniza-tions	2		
Smoking	5	Colorectal screening	4		
Pregnancy	1	Cholesterol	3		
Women's health	10				
HIV/AIDS	14				
Demo-graphics	14				
Total		*Total*	22	*Total*	22
Women	53				
Men	42				

core questions generally stay on the questionnaire for 1 year, although the questions can be extended for an additional year. Since 2000, the BRFSS questionnaire has followed the 1993–2000 plan, although a new plan will likely be developed for the 2005–2015 decade.

A number of criteria were identified in 1995 to guide selection of items for the BRFSS questionnaire. These include the relationship of the variable to personal behaviors linked to promoting health, preventing disease, or reducing health risks; suitability of the question for telephone interviewing; pertinence of the variable to national health objectives or other priority health issues; the need to measure the variable over time; the need to have state-specific data; the degree to which alternative data sources are unsatisfactory; the degree to which the prevalence of the variable will be adequate for planned analyses; the relationship of the variable to other questionnaire topics; and the quality of the measure. Additional criteria include financial and technical resources available for support of the question and the effect on questionnaire length, considering both the total number of questions and the proportion of respondents to be queried.

In addition to administration of the core questionnaire, the BRFSS state coordinator is responsible for determining which, if any, optional modules or state-added questions will be included. The coordinator develops a process for obtaining recommendations from various programs in the state health department that would benefit from data derived from these optional components. Although CDC has supported up to 19 modules annually, it is not feasible for a state to use them all. States are selective in their choices of modules and state-specific questions to keep the questionnaire at a reasonable length (though there is wide variation across states in the total number of questions for a given year, ranging from a low of about 90 to 150 or more). Additional funding for particular modules is also a factor in deciding which modules to include. New questionnaires are implemented in January and usually remain unchanged throughout the year. However, the flexibility of state-added questions does permit additions, changes, and deletions at any time during the year, notably when emerging issues arise.

BRFSS SAMPLE DESIGN

Population

The target population in the BRFSS is the noninstitutionalized civilian population aged 18 years or older in each participating state or territory.

Coverage

Respondents in households are identified through telephone-based methods. Telephone coverage is known to be at least 95% in the U.S., but is lower for some groups, including minorities and those with lower socioeconomic status (U.S. Bureau of the Census, 1994). No direct method of compensating for non-telephone coverage is employed by the BRFSS. Poststratification weights by age/race/sex or age/sex categories are used in the BRFSS, which may partially correct for any bias caused by non-telephone coverage.

BRFSS Samples

The BRFSS surveys in each state and territory employ random digit dialing (RDD) methods of sampling. Specific sampling methods have varied among states, but as mentioned above all now use DSS. Interviews are conducted each month of the year, usually during a 2-week period, and each state has a target number of interviews. For example, in 1999, interviews ranged from about 100 to 425 per month, yielding annual state samples from about 1,200 to 5,100. States that are interested in making estimates for sub-state areas (domains) may sample at different rates in particular strata to ensure a minimum sample size per stratum; these samples are referred to as stratified samples. A number of states used this type of design from the beginning.

Quality Control

During the early years of the BRFSS operation, CDC had sole responsibility for editing the data. However, now all states edit the data before they are sent to CDC for processing. The data currently undergo two additional edit checks at CDC. Furthermore, quality control reports are generated by CDC as the data are received, and results returned to the states for any corrective action that may be necessary. At the end of each year, an annual quality control report is prepared that compares data across states and provides information on response rates.

DATA DISSEMINATION

The Behavioral Surveillance Branch has a policy to provide timely access to BRFSS data to any who request the information. Specifically, the branch provides BRFSS data that have been edited and are ready for statistical analysis with weights and uniform variable formats. Priority is given to participating states for access to their own BRFSS data.

After each state has an opportunity to review their own data, the BRFSS data for all states are made available to others both within and outside CDC, a process which now takes about 3 to 4 months after the end of the data collection year. From the mid to late 1990s, data were made available on CD-ROM; more recently, they can be easily downloaded from the BRFSS Web site, which debuted in 1997 (www.cdc.gov/brfss). In addition to the data, the Web site provides other BRFSS-related information. For example, documentation for the data are available, as well as basic information about the system, survey instruments for most years, summary tables of prevalence estimates, trend data, and lists of BRFSS publications. New items continue to be developed that will be accessible from the Web site, such as an index of questions and selective training modules.

DATA ANALYSIS AND USE

Data Use at the State Level

An important aspect of the BRFSS is how the data are utilized and disseminated within states. Major uses are to estimate the prevalence of important behaviors that contribute to morbidity and mortality, identify demographic variations in health-related behaviors, target programs and services, address emergent and critical health issues, guide health legislation and policy, and measure progress toward state and national health objectives. During the 1990s, a number of topics on the BRFSS were linked to specific objectives set forth in the Healthy People 2000 initiative (U.S. Department of Health and Human Services [DHHS], 1991). Current questionnaires are linked to national health objectives for 2010 (DHHS, 2000). In fact, 7 of the 10 leading health indicators for 2010 can be measured by the BRFSS. Such use of the BRFSS provides state policy makers with informed options for public health decisions. Although use of the BRFSS for decision-making is central at the state level, it is not the exclusive function. BRFSS data assist in designing public-health intervention strategies and evaluating their impact on the state's population.

Disseminating findings is also an important part of the surveillance system. All BRFSS-participating states prepare reports or fact sheets to educate the public, the health professional community, and legislators about the current status and trends in lifestyle patterns in their state. Table 6.2 provides examples of BRFSS data applications at the state level.

Use of BRFSS data to address specific health issues varies from state to state. Currently, all states use BRFSS data to establish and track state health objectives, plan health programs, or implement a broad array of disease prevention activities. Nearly two thirds of states use BRFSS data to support health-related legislative efforts.

For example, BRFSS data have been used to support tobacco control legislation in most states, and particularly in California, where the data were influential in supporting the passage of Proposition 99 Tobacco Tax legislation, which generated millions of dollars in state funds to support health education and chronic disease prevention programs. With passage of the National Breast and Cervical Cancer Mortality Prevention Act by Congress in 1990, funds became available to state health departments to establish breast and cervical cancer control programs. Surveillance data on use of mammography and Pap tests from the BRFSS provide critical information to states about baseline

TABLE 6.2.   Examples of How BRFSS Data Have Been Used by State Health Departments

Guide health policies
Determine priorities and plan long-range strategies
Monitor progress toward state or national health objectives
Guide minority health program initiatives
Monitor the effectiveness of prevention program
Propose and support legislation
Assess and document needs
Develop point-in-time studies
Document state-specific prevalence of selected behaviors
Monitor program goals
Guide educational interventions
Develop community surveys
Increase public awareness
Influence physician adherence
Prepare proposals for funding
Guide resource allocation
Serve as models for other surveys

cancer screening levels and provide a means to monitor breast and cervical cancer control program impact.

In Illinois, two successful legislative initiatives were supported by data on the prevalence of smoking and mammography screening: an act requiring no smoking areas in public buildings and one requiring the inclusion of mammography screening in all health insurance coverage. In Nevada, BRFSS data documenting the state's high rates of chronic and binge drinking were used to support legislation to place a per-gallon tax at wholesale level on distilled alcohol. Cardiovascular disease continues to be the focus of state health promotion and risk reduction efforts because of its tremendous morbidity and mortality burden. The BRFSS data provide a continuous way to monitor changes in cardiovascular-related health behaviors in the population and assess the effectiveness of risk reduction initiatives in many states. Numerous additional examples can be found in a CDC publication that summarizes the results of a survey of state BRFSS programs on how each has used the data (CDC, 2000a).

Data Use at the Federal Level

The task of analyzing data from the BRFSS and encouraging and promoting analysis of the data rests primarily with the Behavioral Surveillance Branch at CDC. Staff are responsible for developing research initiatives, establishing priorities and tracking progress, and consulting or collaborating with state health departments, other centers and divisions within CDC, and organizations outside CDC (other federal agencies, national and international health agencies, voluntary health agencies, and universities), who have an interest in analyzing data from the BRFSS.

Similar to the states, analysis and use of the data at the federal level includes estimating the prevalence of important behaviors that contribute to morbidity and mortality, identifying demographic variations in health-related behaviors, targeting programs and services, addressing emergent and critical health issues, guiding health legislation and policy, and measuring progress toward health objectives. However, because researchers at the federal level have ready access to BRFSS data from all participating states and because more years of data are available (states entered the system at different times), these analyses are often at the regional or national level.

Essentially every topic area covered by the BRFSS has been analyzed and reported from summary reports of each variable across states

(Bolen, Rhodes, Powell-Griner, Bland, & Holtzman, 2000; Holtzman et al., 2000) to reports on a single behavior or practice that contributes to disease or injury (CDC, 2000b; Ebrahim, Floyd, Merritt, Decoufle, & Holtzman, 2000; Li, Serdula, Bland, Nelson, & Mokdad, 2000; Nelson, Grant-Worley, Powell, Mercy, & Holtzman, 1996). To date, there have been well over 500 BRFSS-related publications, and at least four times as many presentations of the data.

Because the BRFSS has been in operation for nearly two decades and many items on the questionnaire have remained unchanged, trends are easily monitored. Numerous reports have looked at BRFSS data over time. One recent example was a publication that examined trends in obesity (Mokdad et al., 1999). In this case, BRFSS data were used to document the growing epidemic of obesity among U.S. adults over the past decade. Another advantage in aggregating the data over place and time (i.e., yielding larger samples) is that select subgroups of the population can be analyzed. For example, older adults (Janes et al., 1999; Mack & Bland, 1999; Powell-Griner, Bolen, & Bland, 1999) or persons of specific race and ethnic groups, such as American Indians and Alaskan Natives, have been examined in several reports (Denny & Taylor, 1999).

Furthermore, because use of optional modules varies by state, scientists can combine states that have used the same modules to obtain larger samples and conduct more in-depth analyses. There are as well numerous examples of publications for many of the BRFSS modules (Holtzman, Bland, Lansky, & Mack, 2001; Saaddine et al., 1999).

International consultation and collaboration is also an activity of the BRFSS. One collaboration involved a BRFSS-type survey in seven municipalities in China. Other countries have also undertaken BRFSS-type surveys, including Russia, Australia, and Canada. Most recently, Brazil and Argentina have consulted CDC about establishing behavioral surveillance for chronic disease and injury.

The extent to which BRFSS data are utilized for state and federal agencies for policy and program development is dependent on the relevance of the data to their needs and the credibility placed in the data as evidenced by reliability and validity. Several studies have been carried out that have examined the reliability or validity of measures on the BRFSS or similar measures from other surveys (Brownson et al., 1999; Martin, Leff, Calonge, Garrett, & Nelson, 2000; Stein, Courval, Lederman, & Shea, 1995). These studies were recently summarized in a paper that covered core BRFSS measures for the years 1993–2000

(Nelson et al., 2001). For measures on the BRFSS that had been studied, most were found to be at least moderately reliable and valid, and several were highly reliable and valid.

LIMITATIONS AND STRENGTHS

Although the BRFSS has experienced marked growth and visibility, there are some limitations. As with many survey systems and especially with large-scale surveillance systems such as the BRFSS, it does not cover any topic in great depth (so as to include as many behaviors related to chronic disease and injury as possible); consequently, there are few items, for example, that measure determinants of behavior. The length of the interview and the increasing competition for space on the BRFSS also constrain the number of questions that can be asked on any one topic. Moreover, even though the system is quite broad, it only covers certain main topics (related primarily to chronic disease and injury), so other areas that one may be interested in researching would have to be found in another system. As a telephone survey, the BRFSS obviously does not include households without telephones and thus most likely underrepresents the nation's indigent population. Nor does it include persons who do not reside in households, such as those who are institutionalized or homeless. Response rates also vary by demographic characteristics. In addition, persons with poor health habits may be more likely to refuse to be interviewed. Further, the data are self-reported and may be subject to under- or overreporting. Finally, the survey is administered in English or Spanish, so those who speak languages other than these would not be included.

Despite these limitations, a system such as the BRFSS offers several advantages. The system is flexible, new questions can be added in a timely manner, and it is relatively inexpensive to operate. Standardized procedures facilitate comparability. States can compare themselves to other states, to a region, or to the nation. Importantly, the system provides prevalence estimates of behaviors that are useful to help evaluate programs and guide legislation. States have their own data on which to base program and policy decisions, yet the data can be easily combined to produce regional or national estimates (*Evaluation of BRFSS*, 1999). Emerging health issues can also be examined in this system. Once established, the system can be adapted for other uses, other topics, other populations, and other countries. For example,

CDC collaborated with the U.S. Air Force to conduct a BRFSS-type survey of Air Force personnel stationed throughout the world (CDC, 1998).

In addition, because many of the same data are collected continuously with a standard methodology, the BRFSS is ideal for monitoring trends. This same structure also allows for a very large amount of data, which enables even small subgroups or low prevalent behaviors within a population to be analyzed and yield relatively stable estimates. Furthermore, the quality of several measures from the BRFSS has been found to be relatively good. Finally, although data from the system can be aggregated to provide national or regional prevalence estimates, in many cases, the BRFSS is the only source of population-based, state-level behavioral data for chronic disease in the United States.

INNOVATION AND CHALLENGES FOR THE FUTURE

Innovation in the BRFSS has occurred at both the state and federal level. In terms of survey administration, most innovation, not surprisingly, occurs at the state level. For example, over time several states moved from in-house interviewing to subcontracting with private corporations. Further, as previously mentioned, all states moved gradually to disproportionate stratified sampling to reduce interviewing costs. In addition, some states have employed oversampling techniques to obtain sufficient numbers for their minority populations, and concurrently developed techniques to adjust their statewide BRFSS estimates for this oversampling. A few states have implemented split-samples to avoid data gaps created by the rotating core. States also have been extremely innovative in designing state-added questions for program and legislative purposes, for example, obtaining information about the level of support for tobacco excise-tax increases. After the bombing of the federal building in Oklahoma City in 1995, the state implemented a special BRFSS-type survey to examine the impact on the emotional and behavioral health of city residents (Smith, Christiansen, Vincent, & Hann, 1999).

At the federal level, innovation generally occurs at the broader procedural level. For example, the concepts of rotating core and emerging questions were developed at the federal level to address the issue of questionnaire length. Standards for data collection and quality assurance are also developed and modified at the federal level. Efforts to enhance the analytic potential and use of the BRFSS data have been primarily a federal initiative. Innovation in electronic dissemination of the data and related information has also been a federal priority. Finally, some innovation has clearly been a joint state-federal venture. One example is the adaptation of the BRFSS for Colorado's Kaiser-Permanente organization; this 1993 activity spurred a collaborative effort among federal and state employees to develop modules and emerging core questions addressing health care access and preventive counseling (Martin et al., 2000). Most recently, CDC is working with the New York BRFSS program to determine how the system might be used to assess the health of adults in New York City in the aftermath of events surrounding the attack on the World Trade Center.

Through the collection of behavioral data at the state level, the BRFSS has proven to be a powerful tool for building health promotion activities. As the system has become more visible and the demand for data has increased, there has been an even greater request from programs within and outside of CDC not only to add questions to the survey, but also to expand data collection beyond the state level. Although the BRFSS was designed to produce state-level estimates, growth in the sample size has facilitated production of smaller-area estimates. To meet the need for prevalence estimates at the local level, data from the 1997 BRFSS were used to calculate estimates for selected urban areas (66 total) in the United States with at least 300 respondents. Preliminary results from this effort showed that the prevalence of certain behaviors varied across cities, not unlike the differences found across states. Variation in prevalence was also observed when cities were compared with their surrounding metropolitan areas and with the rest of the state. These data should help cities to better plan and direct their prevention efforts. Because of the success of this effort, selected city estimates for the years following 1997 have been made or are being planned.

In addition to expansion within the United States, requests continue to increase for technical assistance from other countries that are eager to develop similar surveillance systems. To aid in this effort, the World Health Organization (WHO), which works in collaboration with CDC to promote behavioral surveillance for noncommunicable diseases, is in the process of developing a model surveillance system based on the BRFSS for export to any country.

In the face of changing technology and the greater demand for data beyond the state level, the challenge for the BRFSS will be how to manage effectively this increasingly complex surveillance system, which serves the needs of numerous programs. One major challenge for the BRFSS is how to deal with the decline in response rates. Similar to other telephone surveys, response rates have been declining over the past decade. Median BRFSS CASRO (Council of American Survey Research Organizations) response rates (White, 1983) dropped from 70% in 1994 to 49% in 2000. Participation rates (the percentage of persons reached by telephone who agree to be interviewed) decreased from 84% in 1991 to 51% in 2000. No doubt this decline can be attributed, at least in part, to changes in telephone technology, including telephone answering machines and caller ID. The proliferation of cell phones also has an impact on reaching and interviewing potential respondents. Respondents who are reached through their cell phones may not be in a position (e.g., in the car) to respond to a survey. Other residents may have only cell phones (rather than land lines) and could take their phones and numbers with them if they move to another state. If this situation becomes more common, it will create sampling issues for the BRFSS, which relies on obtaining a sample of adults who reside in a particular state. Competition from telemarketers has also likely impacted the probability of the respondent's answering the phone.

This is just one important issue facing the BRFSS in the new century. Telephone methods may have to be augmented with other types of data collection. Other methods may have to be implemented altogether (e.g., Web-based surveys). This challenge, as well as others that will likely arise in the future, will have to be addressed. Only by working closely with our state and federal partners to resolve these issue can we continue to provide information useful for effective public-health research and practice.

REFERENCES

Anderson, R., Davies, J. K., Kickbusch, I., McQueen, D. V., & Turner, J. (Eds.). (1988). *Health behavior research and health promotion*. Oxford, UK: Oxford Medical.

Bolen, J., Rhodes, L., Powell-Griner, E., Bland, S., & Holtzman, D. (2000, March 24). State-specific prevalence of selected health behaviors by race and ethnicity, Behavioral Risk Factor Surveillance System, 1997. *CDC Surveillance Summaries, Morbidity and Mortality Weekly Report, 49*(SS-2), 1–60.

Brownson, R. C., Eyler, A. A., King, A. C., Shyu, Y. L., Brown, D. R., & Homan, S. M. (1999). Reliability of information on physical activity and other chronic disease risk factors among US women aged 40 years or older. *American Journal of Epidemiology, 149*, 379–391.

Centers for Disease Control and Prevention. (1998). Behavioral risk factors among U.S. Air Force active-duty personnel, 1995. *Morbidity and Mortality Weekly Report, 47*(28), 593–596.

Centers for Disease Control and Prevention. (2000, January). *BRFSS in action: Tracking health objectives.* National Center for Chronic Disease Prevention and Health Promotion, Division of Adult and Community Health, Behavioral Surveillance Branch. Published by (the Behavioral Surveillance Branch at) CDC, Atlanta, GA.

Centers for Disease Control and Prevention. (2000b). Leisure-time physical activity among overweight U.S. adults trying to lose weight, 1998. *Morbidity and Mortality Weekly Report, 49*(15), 326–330.

Denny, C. H., & Taylor, T. L. (1999). American Indian and Alaska Native health behavior: Findings from the Behavioral Risk Factor Surveillance System, 1992–1995. *Ethnicity & Disease, 9*(3), 403–409.

Ebrahim, S. H., Floyd, R. L., Merritt, R. K., Decoufle, P., & Holtzman, D. (2000). Trends in pregnancy-related smoking rates in the United States, 1987–1996. *Journal of the American Medical Association, 283*, 361–366.

Evaluation of the Behavioral Risk Factor Surveillance System (BRFSS) as a source for national estimates of selected health risk behaviors: Final report. (1999). Baltimore: Battelle.

Frazier, E. L., Franks, A. L., & Sanderson, L. M. (1992). Behavioral risk factor surveillance data. In Using chronic disease data: A handbook for public health practitioners (pp. 1–17). Atlanta, GA: Centers for Disease Control.

Gentry, E., Kalsbeek, W., Hogelin, G., et al. (1985). The behavioral risk factor surveys: II. Design, methods, and estimates from combined state data. *American Journal of Preventive Medicine, 1*, 9–14.

Groves, R. M., & Kahn, R. L. (1979). Surveys by telephone: A national comparison with personal interviews. New York: Academic Press.

Holtzman, D., Bland, S. D., Lansky, A., & Mack, K. A. (2001). HIV-related behaviors and perceptions among adults in 25 states, 1997 Behavioral Risk Factor Surveillance System. *American Journal of Public Health, 91*, 1882–1888.

Holtzman, D., Powell-Griner, E., Bolen, J., & Rhodes, L. (2000). State- and sex-specific prevalence of selected characteristics—Behavioral Risk Factor Surveillance System, 1996 and 1997. *Morbidity and Mortality Weekly Report, 49*(SS-6), 1–39.

Janes, G. R., et al. (1999, December 17). Surveillance for use of preventive health-care services by older adults 1995–1997. *CDC Surveillance Summaries, Morbidity and Mortality Weekly Report, 48*(SS-8), 51–88.

Li, R., Serdula, M., Bland, S. D., Nelson, D. E., & Mokdad, A. (2000). Trends in fruit and vegetable consumption among US adults: Behavioral Risk Factor Surveillance surveys in 16 states from 1990 to 1996. *American Journal of Public Health, 90*(5), 777–780.

Mack, K. A., & Bland, S. D. (1999). HIV testing behaviors and attitudes regarding HIV/AIDS of adults aged 50-64. *The Gerontologist, 39*(6), 687–694.

Marks, J. S., et al. (1985). The behavioral risk factor surveys: I. State-specific prevalence estimates of behavioral risk factors. *American Journal of Preventive Medicine, 1,* 1–8.

Martin, L. M., Leff, M., Calonge, N., Garrett, C., & Nelson, D. E. (2000). Validation of self-reported chronic disease and health services data in a managed care population. *American Journal of Preventive Medicine, 18,* 215–218.

McQueen, D. V. (1996). Surveillance of health behavior. *Curr Issues Public Health, 2,* 51–55.

Mokdad, A. H., Serdula, M. K., Dietz, W. H., Bowman, B. A., Marks, J. S., & Koplan, J. P. (1999). The spread of the obesity epidemic in the United States, 1991–1998. *Journal of the American Medical Association, 282,* 1519–1522.

Nelson, D. E., Grant-Worley, J. A., Powell, K., Mercy, J., & Holtzman, D. (1996). Population Estimates of Household Firearm Storage Practices and Firearm Carrying in Oregon. *Journal of the American Medical Association, 275,* 1744–1748.

Nelson, D. E., Holtzman, D., Bolen, J., Stanwyck, C., & Mack, K. A. (2001). Reliability and validity of measures from the Behavioral Risk Factor Surveillance System (BRFSS). *Social and Preventive Medicine* (Supplement), Birkhauser Verlag Press, Basel.

Powell-Griner, E., Bolen, J., & Bland, S. D. (1999). Health insurance coverage and use of preventive services among the near-elderly in the United States. *American Journal of Public Health, 89,* 882–886.

Saaddine, J. B., Narayan, K. M., Engelgau, M. M., Aubert, R. E., Klein, R., & Beckles, G. L. (1999). Prevalence of self-rated visual impairment among adults with diabetes. *American Journal of Public Health, 89*(8), 1200–1205.

Smith, D. W., Christiansen, E. H., Vincent, R., & Hann, N. E. (1999). Population effects of the bombing of Oklahoma City. *Journal of the Oklahoma State Medical Association, 92,* 193–197.

Stein, A. D., Courval, J. M., Lederman, R. I., & Shea, S. (1995). Reproducibility of responses to telephone interviews: Demographic predictors of discordance in risk factor status. *American Journal of Epidemiology, 141,* 1097–1106.

U.S. Bureau of the Census. (1994, July). Phoneless in America. *Statistical Brief.*

U.S. Department of Health and Human Services. (1991). *Healthy people 2000: National health promotion and disease prevention objectives. Full report, with commentary.* Washington, DC: U.S. Department of Health and Human Services, Public Health Service. DHHS publication no. (PHS) 91-50212.

U.S. Department of Health and Human Services. (2000, November). *Healthy People 2010.* 2nd ed. With understanding and improving health and objectives for improving health. 2 vols. Washington, DC: U.S. Government Printing Office.

Waksburg, J. (1978). Sampling methods for random digit dialing. *Journal of the American Statistical Association, 73,* 40–46.

White, A. (1983). Response rate calculation in RDD telephone health surveys: current practices. In: *Proceedings of the American Statistical Association,* Section on Survey Research Methods, Alexandria, VA, 277–282.

Chapter 7

Qualitative Methods in Community-Based Research

Claire E. Sterk and Kirk W. Elifson

One of the main challenges social and behavioral investigators encounter in conducting community-based research is the selection of an appropriate methodological paradigm for their studies. The two main research paradigms commonly used by social and behavioral scientists are either quantitative or qualitative or, less frequently, a combination of the two. Quantitative explorations typically seek to test a theory, which, in turn, often is translated into hypotheses centered around variables that can be operationalized and analyzed using statistical procedures. The quantitative research paradigm can be labeled as positivistically based. The emphasis is on scientific objectivity and the assumption is made that what is "real" can be discovered. In order to discover what is real, the investigators have to build on the knowledge they already have and ask the "right" questions and look for the appropriate relationships as captured in the hypotheses. In addition, real facts are most easily identified if the researcher and those being researched remain distant and if the researcher is in control of the interaction. Questionnaires are a good example of this. Interviewers are instructed to follow a rigid script; not to deviate from the instructions on order, response categories, or skip patterns; and not to explain any questions to the respondent or elaborate on a topic. The nature of the interaction is similar to a clinical interrogation, which is assumed to result in less bias than if the interaction were more equal. In community-based research, questionnaires may cover topics such as community cohesion, community resources, and, for example, perceptions of, and experiences with, violence and crime. A study participant who has encountered violence or who is the victim of crime is allowed to report on this experience only within the constraints of the data collection instrument. If the study participant is agitated, the interviewer may propose a break or perhaps even terminate the interview, and may propose a referral to a social or health service provider upon completion of the interview. Though the facts are being captured, the reality behind these facts remains unknown.

Qualitative inquiries, on the other hand, seek to develop a complex and holistic understanding, often based in the natural setting, from the perspective of the study participants. Rather than assuming objectivity, qualitative researchers are more likely to admit that they bring personal values and scientific interests into the research. They are aware of their values and acknowledge that the reality is subjective. By collecting data in the natural setting, for example, a community-based organization or the person's home, the distance between the researcher and the study participant is reduced. That the interviewer asks open-ended questions is an indication of the role of the study participant as the expert. The nature of the interaction is collaborative and comparable to a dialogue. Power and control are shared.

The quantitative and qualitative paradigms vary along a number of dimensions, as is reflected in the assumptions made in each of the approaches (Creswell, 1994; Firestone, 1987; Guba & Lincoln, 1988). A final area in which the differences between the paradigms are clear is the data analysis. Quantitative studies tend to result in numerical data and the analysis process focuses on statistical connections. In qualitative studies the data tend to be textual and these are analyzed around themes that provide an interpretative understanding. In general, quantitative methods build on the deductive logic in which hypotheses are developed a priori and subsequently tested, the research design—including the sampling frame and data collection—is static, and one in which reliability and validity are central. Qualitative methodologies are guided by induction, theory is developed from the data, the study participants' perspective is central, the research design is dynamic and emerges as the study evolves, and triangulation using multiple sources as a form of data verification is important.

The selection of the appropriate paradigm should be guided by the research questions to be answered and the scope of the study. For example, the quantitative paradigm is ideal when the researchers have a body of knowledge upon which to build; the qualitative paradigm is better suited for exploratory inquiries that focus on the meaning or nature of experiences (Stern, 1980). Small-scale studies with a limited geographical context are more amenable to a qualitative inquiry, whereas quantitative approaches can be utilized with larger and more geographically diverse samples. In addition, the selection of the research paradigm is likely to be partially determined by the preference of investigators as well as their disciplinary background.

In theory, quantitative and qualitative paradigms allow for scientific inquiry and both are valuable. However, it is not uncommon among scholars and the public at large to view quantitative studies as more scientific and to assume that only what can be measured is scientific (Kaplan, 1964). The qualitative paradigm is viewed as less scientific because it largely produces text rather than numbers. This underappreciation of qualitative research is also reflected in the reference to qualitative data studies as anecdotally based. Nevertheless, once a better understanding is gained of the scientific rigor underlying qualitative research and of the insights it provides into people's lives and experiences or cultural phenomena, appreciation for the qualitative paradigm increases.

It is also important to acknowledge that there is a wide range of approaches to doing qualitative research (see, for example, Denzin & Lincoln, 2000; Morse & Field, 1995). Like quantitative methods and statistical techniques that have developed over time, qualitative research has evolved as well during several phases.

Based on shifts in, for example, epistemology, style, and ethics, seven historical moments can be identified (Denzin & Lincoln, 2000). These include the traditional period (1900–1950) during which qualitative researchers tended to use positivist approaches to produce "objective" accounts of exotic cultures (Geertz, 1988; Rosaldo, 1989); the modernist period (1950–1970) during which much emphasis was placed on formalizing qualitative research as well as its use in gaining an understanding of social processes (Glaser & Strauss, 1967; Lofland & Lofland, 1995; Taylor & Bogdan, 1998); the blurred genres period (1970–1986) focuses on representation and the search among qualitative researchers to locate themselves and their subjects in reflexive text (Geertz, 1973, 1983). The distinction between the social sciences and humanities became blurred during this later period. The crisis of representation period (1986–1990) was characterized by the search for new models of truth, method, and representation and the writing become increasingly reflective (Clough, 1992; Rosaldo, 1989). This extended into the postmodern period (1990–1995) of experimental ethnographic writing (Fine et al., 2000) and the postexperimental inquiry (1995–present).

Although the emphasis of qualitative research depended on the historical context in which it was conducted, the following generic definition developed by Denzin and Lincoln (2000, p. 3) captures its essence:

> [q]ualitative research is a situated activity that locates the observer in the world. It consists of a set of interpretive, material practices that make the world visible. These practices . . . turn the world into a series of representations, including field notes, interviews, conversations, photographs, recordings, and memos to the self. At this level, qualitative research involves an interpretive, naturalistic approach to the world.

Qualitative researchers have been compared with *bricoleurs*, quilt makers or persons who assemble images into montages that ultimately result in a film (Becker, 1998; Levi-Strauss, 1966; Nelson, Trencher, & Grosser, 1992; Weinstein & Weinstein, 1991). A recent example of a "montage" of qualitative research is the collection of essays dealing with women who are HIV positive or who have AIDS (Lather & Smithies, 1997). As the authors indicate, "This book is laid out so that, rather than only giving voice to the stories of others, this is also a book about researchers both getting out of the way and getting in the way" (pp. xiii–xiv).

A sound qualitative research design assumes an approach that is simultaneously rigorous and flexible in order to capture the nuances and complexities of the social situation under study (Flick, 1998). Among the major challenges confronted by qualitative researchers is the selection of a strategy of inquiry. The strategies of inquiry are connected to specific methods for data collection. In this chapter we will discuss the following data collection methods: interviewing, focus groups, observation, case studies, and the review of documents. The final section of this chapter will address the analysis of qualitative data.

INTERVIEWING

Interviewing is one of the most widely used forms of data collection and it can include face-to-face individual, dyadic or group interviewing, and telephone surveys. More recently, virtual interviewing has become an option. Interviews can be informal and unstructured or more formal and semistructured or structured. Finally, interviews can involve a one-time event or a series of data collection moments (see, for example, Lincoln & Guba, 1985; Spradley, 1979). The main goal of conducting an interview is for the interviewer to gain knowledge and insight from the respondent. Independent of the use of a quantitative or qualitative inquiry strategy, the interviewer has to be an "interested listener" who does not bias or judge the interviewees' responses (Converse & Schuman, 1974).

The most common form of interviewing varies by research paradigm. In quantitative research, structured interviews are most common. These are interviews based on a questionnaire, consisting of questions presented in a specific order and with predetermined response categories from which the interviewee selects one or more choices. The researchers determine in advance which questions will be posed and which response categories are provided. The inclusion of *other* as a response choice acknowledges that the study participant may wish to provide an answer other than the options provided by the researchers. Sometimes, the questionnaire allows room for recording the actual content of the *other* response. This structured approach to data collection is consistent with the positivistic perspective and creates the impression of the interviewer as distant, neutral, and objective.

The most common forms of interviewing in qualitative research are the semistructured and unstructured interviews. The assumption underlying semistructured and unstructured interviewing is that the study participants are knowledgeable, have a meaningful perspective to offer, and are able to make this explicit in their own words. Consequently, the nature of the interaction between the interviewer and study participant takes on a different meaning than in structured interviews. The interviewer is an active participant and it is essential that rapport be established with the interviewee.

The semistructured interview follows a series of open-ended questions that often are asked in a particular order. Unstructured interviews are centered around a series of open-ended questions or a list of topics to be discussed. The order in which topics are addressed is irrelevant and not all topics may be raised with each respondent. Unstructured interviewing requires the interviewer to have a plan about the general topics to be discussed, but the conversation—the data-gathering process—determines how and when in the dialogue the information is obtained. The results of unstructured and semistructured interviews provide information on the topics and themes that are salient to the study participant, the appropriate language to be used and the meaning of this language, and the various subgroups within the study population, which in turn assists in determining the sampling frame and recruitment strategies. In addition, this type of interviewing allows the interviewer to generate theory because it allows for description and discovery.

A unique form of qualitative interviews is the life history, a clear definition of which seems to be lacking (Schwandt, 1997). Denzin (1989, p. 48) defines a life history as an "account of a life based on interviews and observations." Life histories can include oral histories, autobiography, or life stories (Tierney, 2000, p. 53). Life histories refer to history as well as memory. They can serve as an entryway "through which the author and the reader might understand a culture different from their own" or life histories "may represent a process whereby the researcher and reader come to understand the semiotic means by which someone else makes sense of the world" (Tierney, 1998). Life histories in community-based studies have the potential to provide a longitudinal perspective.

Qualitative interviews are more difficult to conduct than structured interviews because the interviewer must constantly consider the participant's response. The interviewer must probe to stimulate the study participant to provide detailed information. One form of probing involves asking *directive questions* about a specific topic or comment and asking more elaborate, open-ended questions to guide the dialogue. Other forms of probing include repeating the last sentence of the study participant's answer or summarizing the answer as a means of indicating that the interviewer is listening—the echo probe. Finally, probing can include showing an encouraging nonverbal expression, such as when the interviewer nods his or her head; verbally through affirmative noises such as "uh-huh," "yeah," or "right"; or being silent. A few moments of silence frequently allow the study participant time for reflection, especially when contemplating complex questions.

It is through probing that the power differential between the interviewer and the study participant is symbolized, even though the conversation may appear to be one between equals. The emphasis on power differences has been stressed by those concerned with the sex and race or ethnicity of the interviewer (Collins, 1990; Herz, 1997; Oakley, 1981; Reinharz, 1992; Warren, 1988).

In many ways, the various types of interviewing and the appreciation for each reflect the ongoing tension between those preferring the quantitative versus the qualitative paradigm. However, increasingly investigators are ignoring this apparently unresolvable debate and have begun using multimethod approaches of interviewing. This approach enhances the ability to capture the complexities of human beings and their lives.

FOCUS GROUPS

The most common form of a group interview is the focus group, an interview with a small group of people to discuss specific topics during a 1- to 2-hour session. This type of qualitative data gathering involves the simultaneous interviewing of individuals, whereby the emphasis is not on the individual responses but on the interaction between the participants. The ideal size of a focus group ranges between 6 and 12 individuals and the interviewer is referred to as the moderator. Commonly, the participants are a homogeneous group of individuals who do not know each other (Krueger, 1974). All members are experts because they belong to the group under study.

Focus groups as an inquiry strategy emphasize the interaction between the group members rather than the individual perspective (Merton, Riske, & Kendall, 1956) and the goal of focus groups is not to reach a consensus. Instead, the aim is for the participants to reflect on the discussion topics, to present their opinions, and to respond to the comments of other group members. In other words, the focus is on the synergistic group effect (Stewart & Shamdasani, 1990). Upon considering the example of teen pregnancy, some adolescents may emphasize one explanation for having become pregnant—for example, to have a human being to love, while others may stress a different reason such as seeking to maintain a relationship. A discussion about these explanations is likely to provide insight into the salience of the various reasons, their meanings, as well as the tension between various subgroups of teens, for example, those whose partner is involved versus those whose partner is not. This example also touches on the issue of the homogeneity of focus group participants. When conducting focus groups on teen pregnancy, it may be important to have separate groups for male and female adolescents. Too much heterogeneity among focus group participants may stand in the way of data collection.

The collective brainstorming process among focus group participants is disrupted if one or more of the group members dominates the discussion, and a major challenge to the moderator is to ensure that all voices are heard and to prevent distortion of individual opinions due to perceived group pressures. Another challenge encountered by researchers who use focus groups is confidentiality. Though the moderator can ensure confidentiality between him or herself and the participants, confidentiality among the participants is more difficult to guarantee. Increasingly, the latter is being emphasized in consent forms and a presentation of pre-focus-group guidelines.

Focus groups are not new to the social sciences. During the 1920s, focus groups were used to develop questionnaires. Later in the twentieth century, after World War II, focus groups became a popular data-collection tool among marketing researchers; and during the last several decades of the century to the present, focus groups also have been used to design and evaluate prevention and intervention programs (Morgan, 1988, 1998). Focus groups as an inquiry strategy challenge the dominance of individualistic data-collection methods among quantitative as well as many qualitative researchers. Collective testimonies are only gradually becoming recognized as an important contribution, even among qualitative researchers.

At times, the assumption is made that focus groups are very cost-effective and require less time than individual qualitative interviews. However, one should keep in mind that these data-collection strategies serve a unique purpose and provide different data. For example, focus group data reveal group dynamics and collective thinking, whereas individual interviews provide in-depth information from a single perspective. In a controlled experiment, Fern (1982) found that focus groups did not produce significantly more information that in-depth interviews. However, some research has shown that the participation in a group might be perceived as more satisfying and stimulating and less threatening than individual face-to-face interviews by the participants (Morgan, 1998; Wilkinson, 1998).

OBSERVING

Although much of the emphasis in interviewing is on what people *say*, observations focus on what people *do*. Observational techniques largely are part of the qualitative paradigm, but even quantitative investigators may rely to a limited extent on observations. For example, during a street interview, nonverbal responses and comments on the interviewee's actions and gestures may be recorded. In order to observe, the researcher has to be part of the setting and much of the ongoing debate has focused on the question to what extent this presence may change the situation under study (see, for example, Adler & Adler, 1987; Pelto & Pelto, 1978; Wolcott, 1995). The least involved method of observations are "windshield observations" in which the researcher is only marginally involved. The following chapter on a case study using qualitative methods gives a good example of the value of such observations in community studies.

When conducting observations, researchers have to pay attention to their role and the extent to which they will immerse themselves in the group under study. The level of involvement can range from being a distant observer to being a complete participant (Gold, 1997; Werner & Schoepfle, 1987). Others have referred to this as a spectrum of membership roles, including "peripheral" or "active" and "complete" members (Adler & Adler, 1987). Clearly this debate is related to discussions about the reliability and validity of observation data.

Others are less concerned with the observer's role and more with developing a typology of systematic observations, consisting of descriptive, focused, and selective observations (Werner & Schoepfle, 1987). Observation as an inquiry strategy also has been referred to as ethnography or fieldwork (see, for example, Agar, 1986; Lofland & Lofland, 1995; Lofland, 1996; Spradley, 1980; Van Maanen, 1988). The process of conducting observations has been labeled as "subjective soaking" (Ellen, 1984) and the written analysis has been referred to as "thick description" (Geertz, 1973).

In order to be able to observe, the researcher has to identify appropriate settings as well as strategies to gain entrance to these settings (Johnson, 1975; Lincoln & Guba, 1985). While reviewing the literature and exploring settings, the ethnographic fieldwork has started. Ethnographic mapping is ideally suited to make initial decisions about potential study settings, especially since such mapping involves the recording of the physical as well as the social infrastructure of these settings (Sterk, 1999).

Public settings are clearly less difficult to enter than private settings. In addition, researchers can more easily conduct observations in public than in private settings. As a result, much of the debate on observation research in public settings and among vulnerable populations has centered around the ethics surrounding "covert" observations (Berg, 1998). Covert observations may be those in which the observer feigns being a legitimate participant to all or some of those under study or in which the observer deceives those being observed about the nature or purpose of the observations.

Once settings have been identified and access has been mediated, the researcher will have developed some contacts with the gatekeepers. In public settings these are more difficult to identify than in private settings. Gatekeepers may assist the researcher in gaining entry, may prevent entry, or may bias the process to guide the researcher only to certain segments of the setting or population under study. Situations with multiple gatekeepers may require diplomacy to avoid aligning too closely with certain persons or segments (Sterk-Elifson, 1995). Gatekeepers may be formally or self-appointed and may have the interest of the group they represent or their own interest at heart. Ideally, the observer should connect with gatekeepers who are guides as well as informants (Berg, 1998; Sterk, 2000). The mapping and negotiations with gatekeepers allow for the development of the observer's network and as the network expands the researcher is likely to become less dependent on her or his initial contacts. The emphasis shifts to building relationships and rapport, while observing and listening, becoming more focused, and writing extensive observation notes. Clearly, an effective observer is not a silent partner, but rather engages in many informal conversations with members of the group under study. Records of these conversations also become part of the records, often referred to as field notes. The writing of such notes requires specific skills and timing (for more information see Bernard, 1994; Sanjek, 1990).

Overall, observation allows the researcher to collect data that are less based on reactivity than, for example, interview data; it assists in identifying salient research questions, and helps provide insight into the social context in which people operate.

CASE STUDIES

Case studies are another form of inquiry and these involve the systematic gathering of in-depth information about a particular place, person, or event. Case studies are not a data-gathering technique, but rather a methodological approach incorporating multiple methods, including interviewing, observations, and document review (Yin, 1989). Case studies can focus on a single person, even an event in an individual's life, a group or organization, or even a community. The core of case studies is to identify the common as well as unique aspects of the case under study and typically such studies are centered around a limited number of specific research questions. A definition commonly used for case studies is "those in which the researcher explores a single entity or phenomenon (the case) bounded by time and activity (a program, event process, institution or social group) and collects detailed information by using a variety of data collection procedures" (Creswell, 1994, p. 12). The findings of a case study are reported in a case report in which the researcher moves from assembling the raw data to organizing and classifying the data to writing the analytic descriptive narrative, which can be organized around time or themes (Patton, 1990).

Case studies can be intrinsic, instrumental, or collective (Stake, 2000). An *intrinsic* case study aims to provide a more in-depth under-standing—a "thick description" (Geertz, 1973) of a particular case that is of interest to the investigator. Intrinsic case studies are not conducted to develop new theoretical explanations. Examples of such case studies may focus on a specific community program or a community-focused public-health campaign including, for instance, messages on local radio stations and billboards. Intrinsic case studies are limited to one specific case—as opposed to a general phenomenon represented by that case—and such studies do not yield findings that can be generalized.

Instrumental case studies, on the other hand, tend to serve a more supportive role in terms of providing insight into a more generic phenomenon, for example, case studies of a particular community-based organization in order to review similar organizations in general. In such case studies, the actual case primarily serves a supportive role (Berg, 1998).

The third type of case study, *collective case studies*, include a number of cases believed to provide a better understanding of larger number of cases. An example of such case studies are multisite program evaluations (Herriott & Firestone, 1983). One also can refer to these case studies as having different purposes: identity, explanation, and control (White, 1992). They provide an opportunity for a comparative analysis that is not available when limiting one's attention to a single case.

DOCUMENT REVIEW

The review of existing documents frequently is referred to as an unob-trusive measure of textual data. Compared to the data-collection strategies discussed so far it requires the least, if any, involvement of active study participants. Existing records are an unobtrusive indicator of numerous aspects of social life. For example, patients' charts derived from clinical settings may be used to learn about treatment plans and how these change over time; in community studies local media such as newsletters, flyers, and records, including minutes and handbooks from local schools, libraries, religious places, and community-based organizations, provide insight into the local current issues. Documents are an important part of the material culture (Hodder, 1982) and allow for the study of cultural processes.

Documents may include official documentary and actuarial records (Berg, 1998). Documents can be public or private, formal or informal (Lincoln & Guba, 1985). Public archives tend to be designed for investigations by others and often the records are in a standardized form and are systematically arranged. Private records are normally not intended to be viewed by others and may be more candid and less well organized. Sometimes private records become public, even if the original intention was not to share the documents with others. An example of informal private records becoming public are personal memories, and an example of formal records produced for a limited audience becoming public are the recently released tobacco industry documents. The latter includes a wide range of records, including newsletters, minutes of meetings, memos, reports on research findings, audio recordings, photos, videotapes, transcripts of speeches, electronic messages, and other forms of communication.

Actuarial records tend to be available in the public domain under certain conditions. Examples are birth records, marriage certificates, divorce and death records, and credit reports. These records may not be complete, resulting in inaccurate or missing data. For example, a researcher interested in reviewing death certificates to gain insight into the early years of the AIDS epidemic may find that few list AIDS as the cause of death. This may be because AIDS as a syndrome may result in listing a specific disease and not as the cause of death or it may reflect a strategy to avoid disclosing the actual cause of death. This example also shows that while document reviewing is an unobtrusive and nonreactive method of inquiry, the records themselves were reactive, in this case to the emerging threat of a new infectious disease associated with stigma due to its route of transmission. Documents not only provide valuable data, but the investigation of documents also is likely to generate new areas of inquiry that may not have emerged if data collection had been limited to interviews and observations.

DATA ANALYSIS

Until this point, the ideology underlying the quantitative and qualitative paradigms has been addressed as have various qualitative data-collection strategies. With the exception of pictures or films, qualitative data tend to be textual in format. An exciting challenge is to organize these data in a systematic way as a first step in the data analysis process. Due to the flexible nature of the data collection, the analysis process may be approached in one of several ways and typically begins almost simultaneously with the data collection. A strategy commonly used is content analysis, the process through which researchers systematically organize and interpret the text (Berg, 1998). In starting the analysis, one can view the textual data as an object of analysis, the linguistic tradition, or one can view the textual data as a window into human experiences, the sociological tradition (Ryan & Bernard, 2000; Tesch, 1990). It is the latter that will be the focus in this section.

A place to start the qualitative data analysis process is by looking at words. The most simple way to do so is by counting how frequently a word occurs (Weber, 1984). A related method is that of semantic network analysis (Danowski, 1993; Schnegg & Bernard, 1996). Typically, it involves the development of matrices of the use of certain words by each respondent. This method too is based on quantifying the textual data. Taking this process a step further are those who develop cognitive maps or meaning networks of concepts as represented in the data (Carley & Palmquist, 1992; D'Andrade, 1991).

More may be gained by placing the words in context. The *key-words-in-context* (KWIC) technique allows for concordance and typically the investigator will include 30 words prior to and 30 words following the key word (McKinnon, 1993). This type of key word analysis provides initial insights into potentially central themes in the textual database. In addition to the frequency of a word or the context in which a word is used, researchers may develop interpretations from the data. Imagine, for example, reviewing the transcripts about interviews in which respondents were asked to: "Describe your community." In those transcripts, the researchers can look for the use of specific words by the respondents. Let us assume that they are interested in differences between long-term residents and newcomers and that the former were more likely to use words like "used to be," "change," and "deterioration of sense of community," while newcomers mentioned "progress," "advancement" and "building community." The responses indicate the different perspectives between the two groups and hint at the fact that the longtime residents reflect on the past, while the newcomers look forward.

Techniques such as word counting, semantic network analysis, and KWIC are designed to quantify and often serve as a first step in the coding process. At the heart of the coding process is the identification of themes. Themes can be identified using schema analysis, in which the researchers look for shifts in content (Agar & Hobbs, 1985); or grounded theory, involving a line-by-line coding process (Becker, 1998; Charmaz, 1990; Glaser & Strauss, 1967; Lincoln & Guba, 1985; Strauss & Crobin, 1990). In this chapter, we will elaborate on the grounded theory approach.

Other than those who limit themselves to quantification, most qualitative researchers move into the inductive data analysis process that involves using data to identify theoretical insights. A good first step is to review carefully all textual data and to underline key phrases and mark sections in the text by placing "code words" in the margin (Sandelowski, 1995). In order to ensure intercode reliability, most qualitative researchers will encourage that the text analyzed be coded by more than one person (Carey, Morgan, & Oxtoby, 1996). The initial product will be a code list, which becomes part of the code book. The latter includes a description of each code and can be compared to a code book as used by quantitative researchers in which each variable is described. The difference is that code books in qualitative research will continue to develop until the analysis process is complete.

When conducting a grounded theory analysis, the researcher engages in an iterative process of reviewing and coding the textual data, while developing insights typically about concepts that capture various codes or model linking codes that are grounded in the data. Sometimes "in vivo" coding is utilized, meaning the analyst refers to terms and themes identified by the study participants themselves (Strauss & Corbin, 1990). As new codes emerge, the researcher may decide to modify the current data-collection instrument or, if data collection was assumed to be complete, that additional data collection is needed.

Qualitative data analysis does not end with the development of initial codes. The next step after the initial coding—also referred to as open coding (Agar, 1996; Bernard, 1994; Lofland & Lofland, 1995)—is to look for connections between codes, referred to as categories (Miles & Huberman, 1994). Axial coding involves the process of relating categories to their subcategories (Strauss & Corbin, 1990). Because the analysis inquiry centers around categories, the investigator is likely to start developing an organizational scheme or paradigm. Throughout this process, the qualitative data analyst will continue to modify and refine the categories, a process referred to as selective coding. The investigator is now ready to move from description to conceptualization.

Glaser and Strauss (1967), who introduced grounded theory, refer to the process of identifying connections and similarities and differences between themes and categories as the *constant comparison method*. Central to this method is the writing of memos or "memoing," while distinguishing between memos that describe the codes, including records of analytical decisions, and those that refer to theoretical insights (Strauss & Corbin, 1990). These memos become part of the qualitative data set.

The written narrative of a qualitative study is centered around the codes, categories, and themes identified in the data analysis process, and typically direct quotes from the narrative are provided. The selection of appropriate quotes presents a challenge, and qualitative researchers should refrain from including only those quotes that support their main point of view while ignoring negative examples. It is important to keep in mind that while coding is a method to gain insight into the data, it also removes the analysis from the raw data. Atkinson (1992, p. 459) states "every way of seeing is also a way of not seeing."

QUALITATIVE DATA MANAGEMENT AND COMPUTERS

With the introduction of word processors, qualitative researchers were able to move away from writing notes by hand, copying files, color-coding materials, and other manual organizational strategies. Computers allowed for easier storage of textual data, organization of text by using line numbers, and for retrieving text through word searches (Fielding & Lee, 1998). The computer programs do not assist in analyzing the data, but rather assist with the data management. Computers do not comprehend the meaning of the data one puts in the system, be those numerical or textual. Weitzman (2000) points out that qualitative-data-management packages allow the investigator to store, edit, and code the data, to search and retrieve certain segments, to link segments of the data, and to display the data. An in-depth description of the various programs goes beyond the scope of this chapter. Typically, one distinguishes between programs that allow the investigators to retrieve text (e.g., ZyIndex), to manage the text (e.g., Folio Views and Textbase Alpha), to code and retrieve data (e.g., Qualpro), and to build theory based on codes (e.g., AnSWR, ATLAS/ti, QSR NUD*IST, and Ethnograph). There is no easy answer to the question of which software is most appropriate; some qualitative investigators challenge the use of software packages for qualitative data analysis for fear that it will reduce the researcher's familiarity with, and closeness to, the data. Similar to the philosophy among quantitative researchers, one must keep in mind that it is more important to understand the dynamics underlying data analysis than it is to use a software package.

REFERENCES

Adler, P. A., & Adler, P. (1997). *Membership roles in field research.* Newbury Park, CA: Sage.

Agar, M. H. (1986). *Speaking of ethnography.* Beverly Hills, CA: Sage.

Agar, M. H. (1996). *Speaking of ethnography* (2nd ed.). Thousand Oaks, CA: Sage.

Agar, M. H., & Hobbs, J. (1985). How to grow schemata out of interviews. In J. Doughery (Ed.), *Directions in cognitive anthropology* (pp. 413–431). Urbana: University of Illinois Press.

Atkinson, P. A. (1992). The ethnography of a medical setting: Reading, writing and rhetoric. *Qualitative Health Research, 2,* 451–474.

Becker, H. S. (1998). *Tricks of the trade: How to think about your research while you're doing it.* Chicago: University of Chicago Press.

Berg, B. L. (1998). *Qualitative research methods for the social sciences* (3rd ed.). Boston: Allyn & Bacon.

Bernard, H. R. (1994). *Research methods in anthropology: Qualitative and quantitative approaches* (2nd ed.). Walnut Creek, CA: Alta Mira.

Carey, J., Morgan, M., & Oxtoby, M. (1996). Intercoder agreement in analysis of responses to open-ended interview questions: Examples from tuberculosis research. *Anthropology Methods Journal, 8,* 1–5.

Carley, K., & Palmquist, P. (1992). Extracting, representing, and analyzing mental models. *Social Forces, 70,* 601–636.

Charmaz, K. (1990). "Discovering" chronic illness: Using grounded theory. *Social Science and Medicine, 30,* 1161–1172.

Clough, P. T. (1992). *The end(s) of ethnography: From realism to social criticism* (2nd ed.). New York: Lang.

Collins, P. H. (1990). *Black feminist thought: Knowledge, consciousness, and the politics of empowerment.* New York: Routledge, Chapman and Hall.

Converse, J. M., & Schuman, H. (1974). *Conversations at random: Survey research as interviewers see it.* New York: Wiley.

Creswell, J. W. (1994). *Research design: Qualitative and quantitative approaches.* Thousand Oaks, CA: Sage.

D'Andrade, R. (1995). *The development of cognitive anthropology.* Cambridge, MA: Cambridge University Press.

Danowski, J. (1993). Network analysis of message content. In W. Richards & G. Barnett (Eds.), *Progress in communication science* (pp. 197–221). Norwood, NJ: Ablex.

Denzin, N. K. (1989). *Interpretive biography.* Newbury Park, CA: Sage.

Denzin, N. K., & Lincoln, Y. (Eds.). (2000). *Handbook of qualitative research* (2nd ed.). Thousand Oaks, CA: Sage.

Ellen, R. F. (1984). *Ethnographic research.* New York: Academic Press.

Fern, R. N. (1982). The use of focus groups for idea generation: The effects of group size, acquaintanceship, and moderator on a response quality and quantity. *Journal of Marketing Research, 19,* 1–13.

Fielding, N. G., & Lee, R. M. (1998). *Computer analysis and qualitative research.* London: Sage.

Fine, M., Weiss, L., Weseen, S., & Wong, L. For Whom? Qualitative research, representations, and social responsibilities. In N. Denzin & Y. Lincoln (Eds.), *Handbook of qualitative research* (2nd ed., pp. 107–132). Thousand Oaks, CA: Sage Publications, Inc.

Firestone, W. A. (1987). Meaning in method: The rhetoric of quantitative and qualitative research. *Educational Researcher, 16,* 16–21.

Flick, U. (1998). *An introduction to qualitative research: Theory, method and applications.* London: Sage.

Geertz, C. (1973). *The interpretation of cultures: Selected essays.* New York: Basic Books.

Geertz, C. (1983). *Local knowledge: Further essays in interpretive anthropology.* New York: Basic Books.

Geertz, C. (1988). *Works and lives: The anthropologist as author.* Stanford, CA: Stanford University Press.

Glaser, B. G., & Strauss, A. L. (1967). *The discovery of grounded theory: Strategies for qualitative research.* Chicago: Aldine.

Gold, R. L. (1997). The ethnographic method in sociology. *Qualitative Inquiry, 3,* 388–402.

Guba, E. G., & Lincoln, Y. (1988). Do inquiry paradigms imply inquiry methodologies? In D. M. Fetterman (Ed.), *Qualitative approaches to evaluation in education* (pp. 88–115). New York: Praeger.

Herriott, R., & Firestone, W. (1983). Multisite qualitative policy research: Optimizing description and generalizability. *Educational Research, 12*(2), 14–19.

Herz, R. (1997). *Reflexivity in voice.* Thousand Oaks, CA: Sage.

Hodder, I. (1982). *Symbols in action.* Cambridge: Cambridge University Press.

Johnson, J. M. (1975). *Doing fieldwork.* New York: Free Press.

Kaplan, A. (1964). *The conduct of inquiry.* Newbury Park, CA: Sage.

Krueger, R. A. (1994). *Focus groups: A practical guide for applied research* (2nd ed.). Thousand Oaks, CA: Sage.

Lather, P., & Smithies, C. (1997). *Troubling the angels: Women living with HIV/ AIDS.* Boulder, CO: Westview.

Levi-Strauss, C. (1966). *The savage mind* (2nd ed.). Chicago: University of Chicago Press.

Lincoln, Y. S., & Guba, E. G. (1985). *Naturalistic inquiry.* Beverly Hills, CA: Sage.

Lofland, J. (1996). Analytic ethnography: Features, failings, and futures. *Journal of Contemporary Ethnography, 24,* 30–67.

Lofland, J., & Lofland, L. H. (1995). *Analyzing social settings: A guide to qualitative observation and analysis* (3rd ed.). Belmont, CA: Wadworth.

McKinnon, A. (1993). The multi-dimensional concordance: A new tool for literary research. *Computers and the Humanities, 27,* 165–183.

Merton, R., Riske, M., & Kendall, P. L. (1956). *The focused interview.* New York: Free Press.

Miles, M. B., & Huberman, A. M. (1994). *Qualitative data analysis: An expanded sourcebook* (2nd ed.). Thousand Oaks, CA: Sage.

Morgan, D. L. (1988). *Focus groups as qualitative research.* Newbury Park, CA: Sage.

Morgan, D. L. (1998). *The focus group guide book.* Thousand Oaks, CA: Sage.

Morse, J. M., & Field, P. A. (1995). *Qualitative research methods for health professionals* (2nd ed.). Thousand Oaks, CA: Sage.

Nelson, C., Trencher, P. A., & Grosser, L. (1992). *Cultural studies: An introduction.* New York: Routledge.

Patton, M. (1990). *Qualitative evaluation and research methods* (2nd ed.). Newbury Park, CA: Sage, Inc.

Pelto, P. J., & Pelto, G. H. (1978). *Anthropological research: The structure of inquiry* (2nd ed.). New York: Cambridge University Press.

Oakley, A. (1981). Interviewing women: A contradiction in terms. In H. Roberts (Ed.), *Doing feminist research* (pp. 30–61). London: Routledge and Kegan Paul.

Reinharz, S. (1992). *Feminist methods in social research.* New York: Oxford University Press.

Rosaldo, R. (1989). *Culture and truth: The remaking of social analysis.* Boston: Beacon.

Ryan, G., & Bernard, R. (2000). Data management and analysis methods. In N. K. Denzin & Y. Lincoln (Eds.), *Handbook of qualitative research* (2nd ed., pp. 769–802). Thousand Oaks, CA: Sage.

Sandelowski, M. (1995). Qualitative analysis: What it is and how to begin. *Research in Nursing and Health, 18,* 371–375.

Sanjek, R. (1990). *Fieldnotes.* Ithaca, NY: Cornell University Press.

Schnegg, M., & Bernard, H. R. (1996). Words as actors: A method for doing semantic network analysis. *Cultural Anthropology Methods Journal, 8,* 7–10.

Schwandt, T. A. (1997). *Qualitative inquiry: A dictionary of terms.* Thousand Oaks, CA: Sage.

Spradley, J. P. (1979). *The ethnographic interview.* New York: Holt, Rinehart and Winston.

Spradley, J. P. (1980). *Participant observation.* New York: Holt, Rinehart and Winston.

Stake, R. (2000). Case studies. In N. Denzin & Y. Lincoln (Eds.), *Handbook of qualitative research* (2nd ed., pp. 435–454). Thousand Oaks, CA: Sage Publications, Inc.

Sterk, C. E. (1999). *Fast lives: Women who use crack cocaine.* Philadelphia: Temple University Press.

Sterk, C. E. (2000). *Tricking and tripping: Prostitution during the era of AIDS.* Putnam Valley, NY: Social Change Press.

Sterk-Elifson, C. E. (1995). Determining drug use patterns among women: The value of qualitative research. In E. Lambert & R. Ashbury (Eds.), *Qualitative methods in drug abuse and HIV research* (NIDA Monograph, pp. 65–83). Washington, DC: Government Printing Office.

Stern, P. N. (1980). Grounded theory methodology: Its uses and processes. *Image, 12,* 20–23.

Stewart, D. W., & Shamdasani, P. M. (1990). *Focus groups: Theory and practice.* Newbury Park, CA: Sage.

Strauss, A. L., & Corbin, J. (1990). *Basics of qualitative research: Grounded theory procedures and techniques.* Newbury Park, CA: Sage.

Taylor, S. J., & Bogdan, R. (1998). *Introduction to qualitative research methods: A guidebook and resource.* New York: Wiley.

Tesch, R. (1990). *Qualitative research: Analysis types and software tools.* New York: Falmer.

Tierney, W. F. (2000). Undaunted courage: Life history and the postmodern challenge. In N. K. Denzin & Y. Lincoln (Eds.), *Handbook of qualitative research* (2nd ed., pp. 537–553). Thousand Oaks, CA: Sage.

Tierney, W. G. (1998). Life history's history: Subjects foretold. *Qualitative Inquiry, 4,* 49–70.

Van Maanen, J. (1988). *Tales of the field: On writing ethnography.* Chicago: University of Chicago Press.

Warren, C. A. B. (1988). *Gender issues in field research.* Newbury Park, CA: Sage.

Weber, R. (1984). Computer-aided content analysis. *Qualitative Sociology, 7,* 126–147.

Weinstein, D., & Weinstein, M. A. (1991). Georg Simmel: Sociological flaneur bricoleur. *Theory, Culture and Society, 8,* 151–168.

Weitzman, E. (2000). Software and qualitative research. In N. K. Denzin & Y. Lincoln (Eds.), *Handbook of qualitative research* (2nd ed., pp. 803–820). Thousand Oaks, CA: Sage.

Werner, O., & Schoepfle, G. M. (1987). *Systematic fieldwork: Vol. 1. Foundations of ethnography and interviewing.* Newbury Park, CA: Sage.

White, H. (1992). Cases are for identity, for explanation, or for control. In C. Ragin & H. Becker (Eds.), *What is a case? Exploring for foundations of social inquiry* (pp. 83–104). Cambridge: Cambridge University Press.

Wilkinson, S. (1998). Focus groups in feminist research: Power, interaction, and the co-construction of meaning. *Women's Studies International Forum, 21,* 111–125.

Wolcott, D. L. (1995). *The art of fieldwork.* Walnut Creek, CA: AltaMira.

Yin, R. (1989). *Case study research: Designs and methods.* Newbury Park, CA: Sage, Inc.

Chapter 8

HIV/AIDS PREVENTION: A CASE STUDY IN QUALITATIVE RESEARCH

Kirk W. Elifson and Claire E. Sterk

An overview on qualitative research is provided in the previous chapter. In addition to the general principles underlying this paradigm, it includes a description of the various data collection strategies, including in-depth interviewing, conducting focus groups, observing, and reviewing documents. In this chapter, we will present a case study that captures the central elements of the qualitative research paradigm as well as the various strategies of inquiry. The case to be presented is the Health Intervention Project (HIP), a community-based HIV-risk-reduction intervention targeting uninfected African American female crack cocaine users. First some background on women, drug use, and HIV/AIDS will be provided.

The unique circumstances of women largely have been ignored in addiction and drug use as well as HIV/AIDS investigations. Initially, women were ignored and later were included as a comparison group to male users (File, 1976; Sutter, 1976). Nevertheless, since the 1970s, women increasingly have been enrolled in addiction studies (Adler, 1975; Chasnoff, 1988; Goldstein, 1979; Inciardi, Pottieger, & Lockwood, 1993; Johnson et al., 1985; Kearney, Murphy, & Rosenbaum, 1994; Lieb & Sterk-Elifson, 1995; Rosenbaum, 1981; Sterk, 1999a). As a result, knowledge unique to women has been discovered. For example, the pathways to drug use tend to vary between men and women. Studies focusing on the initiation into drug use have shown that initial drug use often occurs in the company of others. Typically, women are introduced to drugs by either a girlfriend or by a male friend, who often is also her sex partner (Rosenbaum, 1981; Sterk, 1999a). Research findings also indicate that the transition from initial to continued use and dependence tends to develop faster among women than among men (Sterk, 1999a).

Since the onset of the AIDS epidemic, a multitude of studies have explored risk factors for HIV infection among drug users, specifically those who inject drugs (DesJarlais, Friedman, & Strug, 1986). Among the risk behaviors identified are the sharing of syringes and other injection paraphernalia such as water, cookers, and cotton; the frequency of drug injections, and the setting of use. In addition to the specific injection risks for HIV transmission, several sexual risk behaviors were identified such as unprotected sex with high-risk sex partners, having multiple partners, and having negative attitudes toward condom use (Booth, Koester, Brewster, Wiebel, & Fritz, 1991; Bux, Lamb, & Iguchi, 1995; Chitwood, Inciardi, & McBride, 1991; Cohen, Navaline, & Metzger, 1994; Compton, Lamb, & Fletcher, 1995; King et al., 1994; Siegel, Falk, Carlson, & Wang, 1995). Most of our current knowledge regarding HIV infection among injection drug users is based upon epidemiological studies, with few ethnographic studies emphasizing the meaning of risk behaviors—primarily the sharing of syringes and other injection paraphernalia—in the social context in which these occur (Booth, Kwiatkowski, & Stephens, 1998; Carlson, Wang, Siegel, Falk, & Guo, 1994; Latkin, Mandell, Vlahov, Oziemkowska, & Celetano, 1996; Ouellet, Jiminez, & Johnson, 1991).

With the emergence of the crack cocaine epidemic in the United States in the 1980s, sexual activity related to crack cocaine use was identified as a risk factor for HIV infection (Chiasson et al., 1991; Chitwood et al., 1991; Edlin et al., 1994; Inciardi et al., 1993; Ratner, 1993; Sterk, 1988). The transmission due to unsafe sex is more likely to pose a risk for women because the exchange of sex for crack is more common among women than among men, and the probability of male to female transmission is higher than that from females to males. Exchanging sex for crack tends to involve unprotected sex with multiple sex partners, many of whom are not known to the women and may be at risk for HIV and other STDs (McCoy & Inciardi, 1993; Sterk, 1999a; Sterk, 2000). The female's male sex partners, including their steady, casual nonpaying and casual paying partners, tend to be the dominant partner in the relationship, thereby making the negotiation of safe behaviors often difficult for women (Deren, Tortu, & Davis, 1993; Kane, 1991), sometimes even placing her at risk for verbal and physical abuse (Boyd, 1993).

Among the key factors associated with sexual HIV risk among women are partner and relationship issues (Fullilove, Fullilove, Bower, Haynes, & Gross, 1990; Kane, 1991; Tortu, Beardsley, Deren, & Davis, 1994), poverty (Amaro, 1988), cultural issues (Thomas & Quinn, 1991), beliefs and attitudes toward condom use (O'Leary, Goodhart, Jemmott, Boccher-Lattimore, 1992), and personal characteristics such as self esteem (Nyamathi & Lewis, 1991).

Findings from prevention intervention studies show the extent of sexual risk reduction among drug users to be more limited than the level of drug-use-related risk reduction (Booth, Kwiatkowski, & Chitwood, 2000; Cottler et al., 1998). Research among women in methadone treatment revealed that women who received skills training were more likely to use a condom and talk about safe sex (El-Bassel & Schilling, 1992). Other studies involving women showed that a social cognitive theory intervention combining risk education with skill building resulted in increased intentions of condom use (DiClemente & Wingood, 1995; Jemmott & Jemmott, 1992). There is a clear need for gender- and culture-specific studies that focus on women (Amaro, 1995; Mays & Cochran, 1988; O'Leary, 1999; Singer, 1991).

Generally, HIV prevention intervention efforts have been based on psychosocial theoretical frameworks such as the health belief model (Rosenstock, 1974; Rosenstock, Strecher, & Becker, 1988), the theory of reasoned action (Azjen & Fishbein, 1977), the social learning theory (Bandura, 1977), and the stages of change theory (Prochaska & DiClemente, 1983; Prochaska, DiClemente, & Norcross, 1992). Although these theoretical frameworks each have contributed to the development of effective interventions, the underlying dynamics tend to focus on the individual and not on the individual in context. In addition, these theories are not derived from the perspective of the members of the target population and gender is not taken into consideration. In HIP, we conducted formative research in order to develop a risk reduction intervention based on information grounded in the experiences of the women who were members of the target group.

FORMATIVE RESEARCH FOR HIP

For the most part, the formative research utilized a qualitative research paradigm, including observational data collection, conducting in-depth interviews, focus groups, and document review. The quantitative data collection involved survey interviews covering topics such as demographic characteristics, medical and reproductive history, drug use and treatment history, psychosocial measures (e.g., self-esteem, self-efficacy, sensation seeking, and impulse control), and household composition and structure. Using a matrix, initial assessments of sexual activity and drug use also were included.

The main goal of the formative research was to gather data that would assist us in developing an appropriate intervention, in terms of both format and content. A qualitative approach ensured that we would emphasize the women's perspective, place their actions in the context in which these occurred, address the women's wide range of social roles—beyond being a crack cocaine user or a woman at risk for HIV infection—and the ways in which the women negotiated their social roles. Rather than testing hypotheses, we wanted to discover and develop an intervention that was grounded in the data as opposed to validating an existing theory (Blumer, 1969; Geertz, 1973; Strauss & Corbin, 1990).

Identifying Places and People: Observing and Ethnographic Mapping

One of the first decisions to be made involved the selection of the target neighborhoods for HIP. We did this through a process of community identification referred to as ethnographic mapping (Sterk, 1999b; Tashima, Crain, O'Reilly, & Sterk-Elifson, 1996). As a first step we reviewed the local epidemiological indicators of HIV/AIDS and crack cocaine, including data from local emergency rooms as reported in the Drug Abuse Warning Network (DAWN), pretrial detention centers as reported in the Arrestee Drug Abuse Monitoring project (ADAM), treatment centers as reported by the Georgia Department of Public Health, and local law enforcement. This information was supplemented with data from local HIV/AIDS and drug researchers involved in cross-sectional and longitudinal survey studies as well as qualitative investigations. Based on this information, we were able to identify various zip codes in which HIV/AIDS and drug use appeared problematic. We opted for the selection of the zip code in which the HIV/AIDS and crack cocaine prevalence and incidence was highest.

To learn more about the various communities within the zip code, we interviewed professional experts who directly interact with drug users and with other people at risk for HIV/AIDS. These included social and health service providers and law enforcement officials. We also conducted expert interviews with individuals such as local educators, religious and political leaders, and property and store owners whose experience made them knowledgeable about the community. These interviews tended to be brief—20 to 30 minutes or less—often were conducted over the phone and focused on general topics such as locations known for crack cocaine use; demographic and other characteristics of crack cocaine users, specifically women; the presence of subgroups of female crack cocaine users; and any other pertinent information. All interviewees also were asked to submit any written documentation their agency or organization had developed regarding drugs, HIV/AIDS, or the community in general, for example, research data, reports, minutes of public meetings, brochures, and newsletters.

In addition to these formal expert interviews, we conducted mapping, using windshield surveys. These observations focused on the physical structures, the nature of the physical resources, the mapping of specific sites such as stores, businesses, schools, religious sites, graffiti, and vacant lots by block; also the social infrastructure such as the nature of gathering places, interactions between people, the nature of activities, and changes in atmosphere over time. This mapping process allowed us to identify places relevant for our research as well as to develop initial contacts in the community, while establishing ourselves as researchers.

In doing the observations, we also were able to begin developing relationships with those more directly involved with drugs, including members of the local crack-cocaine scene. Informal interviews or interactions with drug users allowed us to gain additional insights and also to develop initial contacts with so-called key informants. Among the key informants were current and former users and dealers. Some key informants proved to be extremely knowledgeable of the local crack-cocaine scene. More common were those who had expertise regarding a small segment of the scene they belonged to or had belonged to, or who served as gatekeepers to a segment. For example, one dealer provided detailed information about the local scene and was able to refer us to a number of crack cocaine users. As we learned more about the community, we realized his description of the scene was relatively accurate, but he failed to provide details of his own role and most of the referrals did not include any of his clients. One woman tried to determine which person in her drug network we should talk with, sometimes providing those we interviewed with her interpretations of the project and what she thought we should hear. These informal expert interviews were conducted at a variety of community settings, lasted about 45 minutes, and were conducted face-to-face.

This process of ethnographic mapping allowed for the comparison of information from local epidemiological indicators, the informal and formal interviews, and our observations, thereby allowing us to triangulate the data and to begin developing an initial plan for targeted sampling (Carlson et al., 1994; Watters & Biernacki, 1989). As part of the targeted sampling, snowball or chain referral sampling assumes the referral to other users. Chain referral sampling allows for the selection of the next study participant through the inclusion of all referrals or the random selection of one of the referrals. Based on the hidden nature of the crack cocaine scene, we opted for a convenience sample of all those who were referred. In other words, each eligible woman would be asked to refer us to other women or to refer these women to HIP, without implementing a randomization process for selection among the referrals. In addition, we assured the initiation of chains in different groups, thereby allowing us to learn about numerous (multiple distinct) social networks (Kaplan, Korf, & Sterk, 1986).

Once we developed a sense of the places and people as well as how the places and the people changed over time—by hour of the day, day of the week, and week of the month—we began more systematic in-depth interviews with female crack-cocaine users and moved from formative and exploratory observations to more structured ones. At that time, we also established the official HIP field site (HIP house) at a centrally located public-housing community within the zip code. We occupied a three-bedroom unit, that also included a living room, kitchen, and bathroom. For a variety of reasons we moved from this unit to a three-bedroom house in the same community. Being in the community but not in public housing offered several advantages, such as being less closely aligned with the public housing community, including its local leaders in the housing association, and becoming more integrated into the community at large. The new HIP house made us neighbors among neighbors. The layout allowed it to become a research field site as well as a safe house where women could come for comfort, clothes, food, or a place to rest and use the facilities.

In-depth Interviews

The in-depth interviews with female crack users were conducted at the HIP house. We conducted a total of 45 interviews, the average length of which was 2 hours. Women were recruited by indigenous outreach workers who were familiar with the community or the drug scene or both (see Sterk, 1999b). Prior to conducting the interviews, all women received a detailed explanation of the formative phase of the study and were asked to sign an informed consent indicating their voluntary participation. The first part of the interview was close-ended and, as mentioned earlier, covered domains such as demographic, psychosocial, sexual, and drug use characteristics. Upon completing this section, the interviewers emphasized open-ended questions and explained to the study participants the importance of feeling free to talk, share their knowledge, and elaborate. The main goal, they explained, was for us as researchers to learn from the women (for more information on qualitative interviewing see chapter 7 on qualitative research). All in-depth interviews were audiotaped and transcribed in preparation for the data analysis. The data analysis followed the constant comparison method, common in grounded theory.

"Pure" qualitative research assumes that the investigators conduct interviews with no predetermined questions or even themes in mind. In reality, however, this seldom is the case, especially if a substantial amount of literature or other information is already available on the topic or target population. Hence, we strived to find a balance between relevant topics as identified in the literature and our own previous research, while also leaving room for the women in HIP to add new topics.

For example, the previous studies indicated that the extent to which women engage in high-risk sex varies (e.g., not using a condom, not being selective in choosing a partner, or engaging in high-risk sex acts), depending on the nature of the relationship between the partners (e.g., length of time the partners have known each other, abuse between the partners, and level of commitment to the relationship) and the setting in which the sexual activity occurs (e.g., drug use versus non-drug-related setting). In addition, researchers have shown that women are at higher risk if they are high on drugs or are experiencing craving or withdrawing and if they use drugs in complex settings (e.g., a setting in which multiple drugs are used or in which users and non-users gather). Gender-related power differences have been identified as largely influencing HIV risk-taking among women. Because of the limited power allocated to women, they often are the "weaker" party in negotiations regarding behaviors. The women's actual and perceived risk for violence and abuse has been reported to function as a barrier to HIV risk reduction.

In addition to gender-specific factors, cultural factors are important. Research has shown that normative beliefs may be mediated by race (Mays & Cochran, 1988; Singer, 1991). Studies involving African American women revealed that they expect men to make decisions related to sexual activity (Fullilove et al., 1990; Worth, 1990) and often view initiating conversations about AIDS with their sex partner as inappropriate. Finally, social support has been associated with perceived capability and actually negotiating HIV risk reduction among women in drug treatment (El-Bassel & Schilling, 1992). Others also have identified social support with HIV protective behaviors (Neaigus et al., 1994). Knowing that others are available for support enhances the women's self-esteem, reduces depression and anxiety, and tends to make them feel more confident about their problem-solving skills.

Thus, examples of the topics covered in the in-depth interviews include a review of the women's childhood and adolescent years, their friendships and (dating) relationships, their medical history (including physical and mental health, drug treatment, and HIV testing), their experiences with drugs (including drug use patterns, changes over time, use by set and setting, and many other details), their sex lives (including the overlap between drug use and sexual activity), social networks and social support, and expectations for the future. Reproductive decision making appeared less salient in the women's account and it was mainly addressed when discussing motherhood. The most prominent emerging themes were the multitude of social roles the women occupied in life, their past and current experiences with violence and abuse, and their ambivalence about changing certain behaviors. Regarding the multiple social roles, the women made it clear that in addition to being crack cocaine users, they also occupied several other important social roles such as being a mother, partner, friend, colleague, and neighbor. They emphasized the importance of being treated as whole human beings and not as "crackheads." From their violence and abuse experiences, we learned that almost all women had either directly or indirectly encountered violence and abuse and that this very much shaped their current realities.

We did not initially ask the women about being African American, but incorporated it as part of the probes. In this regard, many women referred to the history of African American women in American society. They stressed that African American women more than White women had a history of having to be independent caregivers. They also talked about the role of African American women in the lives of White families, for example, by working as a maid or child caretaker. Other issues mentioned were the importance of the extended family as a source of social support to African American women, the use of religion and spirituality as a coping strategy, and the frequent, at times subtle, experiences with racism.

Findings for Intervention Content

Based on the in-depth interviews, we learned the following lessons for the content of the intervention. It would be important to present the HIV/AIDS epidemic and information about the crack cocaine scene at the local level. Data on national, regional or even city-wide trends were perceived as too abstract. We also realized that even though our main (research) goal was to assist the women in reducing their risk for becoming infected with HIV, this might not necessarily be their priority. Hence, it became clear from the formative research that in order to address HIV risk reduction, we needed to sensitize the women to its importance and help them identify their priorities. As a result, we needed to discuss priority-setting in general. For example, a woman would be asked to list her priorities for making changes in her life. Often these included wanting to reduce or give up drugs, to develop a healthy relationship, to be a loving and caring mother, to have a job, and to own a house in a neighborhood with more physical and social resources than her current neighborhood. Some would mention HIV/AIDS, others would not. Among the latter, we initiated a dialogue about what it would take to make HIV risk reduction a priority.

Another lesson involved the importance of assisting women in setting realistic and specific expectations. For instance, establishing a happier life in a healthier environment was a desire expressed by most women. However, when asked about their expectations for the future, these goals often appeared unrealistic. One example that emerged with frequency was a desire to become a registered nurse. However, for many this meant they would have to spend years on their education, at times starting with getting a GED. As the women began to understand what would be required to achieve their expectation, many realized it was more than they had considered or maybe even were willing to do. The formative research showed that by assisting women in setting realistic expectations, they were less likely to encounter disappointments, but rather would experience successes, which in turn would enhance their self-esteem and hope for future accomplishments.

As part of this process, women also brought to our attention that it is important to know what price one is willing to pay. For example, when talking about sex with a steady partner, many women revealed that they preferred not to use a condom because it would be seen as a sign of distrust, would create distance, or would reflect their sexual encounters with paying partners or those who traded sex for crack. By presenting an intervention that encouraged women always to use a condom with a steady partner, we would not respect their "bottom line" regarding sex with steady partners. Instead, the intervention would gain from addressing the notion of this bottom line. Finally, many women emphasized the importance of a referral system to social and health services that were respectful of them as women. Many had negative experiences with service providers who began treating them differently immediately upon learning they were drug users.

We eventually designed two distinct enhanced intervention conditions, using available models that had proven successful with drug users or women but adding the wealth of information from the in-depth interviews. One of these conditions focused on motivation and stressed learning to set priorities along with addressing the women's ambivalence regarding change. The second enhanced condition emphasized negotiation or conflict resolution.

Findings for Intervention Format

The in-depth interviews also revealed information pertinent to the format of the intervention. A key finding was the importance of the site at which the intervention was delivered. The women stressed that the project should be located in their community, should be open only to women, and should not just be a place for research but also a safe place to escape from daily hassles or to find a moment to rest. In other words, it was their place as much as ours. This meant that we had to negotiate with the women how to balance our research needs with their needs; that we needed to explain to the men in the community why they could not enter the HIP house; and that we wanted the women not only to take figurative ownership, but also to take on active roles such as helping with the food and clothing bank we provided, serving as community liaisons, and becoming ex officio members of the research team.

The women had access to the HIP House; however, they were not allowed to stay overnight, and restrictions were placed on their use of the kitchen, bathroom, and other facilities related to the research. We did open the HIP house for activities that were not directly related to the research purposes, with community barbeques—sometimes accompanied by the DJ of a favorite radio station—being the most popular.

Another key finding regarding the content of the intervention involved the nature of the sessions. Many women indicated that the interview was the first time they had spoken to someone openly about their lives, including their abuse experiences (one half had such experiences) and reflecting on their future. This taught us that as intervention researchers, we should be extremely careful not to act as if we were also psychiatrists, psychologists, social workers, or any expert the women needed. Instead, we needed to clarify our role and explain our referral strategy. We also learned during the in-depth interview of the need for initial individual intervention sessions. The private nature of an individual session was expressed as more appropriate and desirable than group sessions. On the other hand, group meetings were favored by the women as a follow-up strategy. As part of HIP, we did deliver individual-level sessions, but we limited group meetings to social events as opposed to intervention sessions. A popular working social event were the reunions for HIP graduates.

Focus Groups

As we moved closer to developing the actual intervention and the manuals for implementation, we conducted a number of focus groups. The first focus group included local HIV/AIDS and drug use experts and we sought their feedback on the preliminary development of the intervention. We learned that many experts agree that an individualized approach to risk reduction is extremely important, but that limited resources precluded a one-on-one approach. On the one hand, we received encouragement for our tailored approach, and on the other we were cautioned. We found that many experts view crack cocaine users as a "hopeless" target group that presented limited possibilities for change. Some experts suggested that we conduct urine analysis to verify a woman's drug use status. After contemplating this suggestion, we opted not to do so. A final key area in which the expert focus group was instrumental was the development of an appropriate referral system.

In addition, we conducted four focus groups with women—two with women who fit the criteria for the HIP target population, one with HIV-negative women from the community who did not use drugs, and one with HIV-positive crack cocaine users. These focus groups validated many of the findings from the in-depth interviews and placed the interview data in context. The women in the non-use focus group expressed their disdain for crack users, but also explained how difficult it was for a woman to be successful in the community once she became an addict. They stressed the importance of role-playing as part of the intervention. The HIV-positive women focused on their past and how important it was to target HIV-negative women. They also emphasized the importance of adequate HIV counseling and testing, with a specific focus on what happens while waiting for test results. In addition, they encouraged us to focus more on communication than on technical skills for HIV risk reduction. In other words, it is okay to teach women how to use a condom or dental dam, but it is more important to teach them to talk about sex and protection.

The two focus groups with HIV-negative women who used crack cocaine confirmed the heterogeneity among female crack-cocaine users in addition to the tension between the various groups. For example, women who did not barter sex for crack were disdainful of those who did; women whose first illicit drug use involved crack looked down on those who in their past had used other drugs, including injected drugs; and those who had lost custody of their children envied those with a social support system that allowed them to hold on to their offspring. These groups also revealed something that was not apparent from the individual interviews, namely the women's ambivalence regarding change. It was in these groups that we learned about the potential resistance to change, their fear of dealing with the consequences of proposing change, the backlash of having failed to implement change, and the importance of explicitly acknowledging their goals for change. Without having had the opportunity to observe the interactions between the women, we would have underestimated the importance of this theme.

Process Interviews and Observations

The qualitative research did not end once the formative phase was completed. We continued our qualitative inquiry as the intervention went on by conducting in-depth interviews with women who had completed the intervention and by continuing the ethnographic mapping. The latter was important to detect changes in the community, including the drug use scene. For example, as HIP evolved, the community underwent a number of changes. The area increasingly became labeled as dangerous and police activity increased, thereby driving the drug scene further underground. In addition, urban slum lords from outside the community discovered the area. They bought available properties very cheaply, renovated the houses with minimum investment, and rented the property for exorbitant amounts. The rent we paid for the HIP house was an example of this new form of entrepreneurship. Local churches—almost every other block in the area had a church or church storefront—decided that the capital should remain in the community and encouraged their members to contribute to the church and the community by renovating houses, for little or no pay, that had been acquired by the church. This process of "urban renewal" changed the community dynamics by creating two classes of residents: those who could afford and those who could not afford to live in renovated housing. In addition, it provided justification for some mobilization against drug users, thereby further marginalizing them.

Our observations and mapping also allowed us to stay informed of changes on the local drug market and the local use patterns. For example, a segment of the neighborhood became known as the city's main heroin distribution point, and over time we saw an increasing number of White persons enter this largely African American neighborhood to buy heroin. Some drug dealers, challenged by a locally saturated crack-cocaine market, began encouraging their clientele to use heroin by providing free samples and teaching people how to smoke crack and heroin simultaneously or how to snort heroin to come down from a crack high (Sterk, 1999a). These new marketing strategies resulted in changes in local drug-use patterns, which we needed to be attuned to in our intervention.

The other continued qualitative inquiry involved open-ended interviews with two types of former participants: those who completed the intervention and those who dropped out. Women who did not complete the intervention attributed it to several causes, including an escalation in their use, the arrest of a boyfriend or their own arrest, a court-ordered admission to drug treatment; or to more positive reasons such as having relocated to a less drug-infested neighborhood or to having secured employment. The in-depth interviews with those women who graduated provided us with excellent process-evaluation information. As part of the data collection specific to the intervention outcomes, women were interviewed 6 months after their graduation from the intervention. However, outcome data were collected using a standardized instrument, leaving little room for learning about the meaning of any behavioral change or the impact of the intervention in general on the lives of the women. A major finding of the process-evaluation interviewing, which followed closely behind the qualitative interviews, was that the survey data only provided a snapshot of the women's behaviors during the 6-month interval, but not on the processes surrounding the complexities of behavioral change. For example, a woman might have reduced her drug use to a limited extent, but she may have consciously gotten high with a select group or at select locations, excluding those in which sexual activity occurred. Though her drug habit might not have changed significantly, her HIV risk was reduced.

Another key finding from these interviews involved the impact of the intervention. Many women mentioned that the areas of HIP that had most influenced their lives were not focused around sexual and drug-related HIV risk, but in gaining a different level of respect for themselves, in learning there are options in their lives, and in realizing that they can take charge of their lives. A response that continued to surprise us was that many women referred to their HIP involvement as an initial step to becoming reintegrated into mainstream society. The key first step for many was our encouragement for them to get a picture ID, and it was amazing how many doors opened with such an ID. For example, many women mentioned that it allowed them to apply for Medicaid.

CONCLUDING REMARKS

The value of employing the qualitative research paradigm is shown in this case study chapter. The various methods utilized are discussed in more detail in the previous chapter on qualitative methods. The qualitative, formative stage of HIP allowed for the development of an intervention that was tailored to the needs of the women targeted in the intervention. The qualitative inquiry methods—focus groups and in-depth interviews—allowed the women's voices to be heard and also facilitated their guiding us as we designed the intervention. Quantitative approaches would have reduced the extent to which the women had input on the intervention development and would not have allowed them to become experts on the research team.

As part of the inquiry, other experts were included as well, for example, community leaders and residents. Their views and experiences assisted the team in gaining a better understanding of the social environment in which the women were functioning, and their vantage point complemented that of the women. The observations provided additional insights on the physical and social infrastructure; reviews of local media, "archives" of community-based organizations, and other written sources further enhanced our understanding.

Once the intervention was underway the inclusion of process observations and interviews allowed for a continued update of our understanding of the women's lives. It also assisted us in guiding the quantitative analysis, for example, by designing composite variables that were grounded in the qualitative data or by helping us define what "risk" and "risk reduction" meant from the women's perspective.

REFERENCES

Adler, F. (1975). *Women in crime.* New York: McGraw-Hill.

Amaro, H. (1988). Considerations for prevention of HIV infection among Hispanic women. *Psychology of Women Quarterly, 12,* 429–443.

Amaro, H. (1995). Love, sex, and power: Considering women's realities in HIV prevention. *American Psychologist, 50*(60), 437–447.

Azjen, I., & Fishbein, M. (1977). Attitude-behavior relations. *Psychology Bulletin, 84,* 888–918.

Bandura, A. (1977). Self-efficacy. *Psychology Review, 84,* 191–215.

Blumer, H. (1969). *Symbolic interactions.* Englewood Cliffs, NJ: Prentice-Hall.

Booth, R., Koester, S., Brewster, J., Wiebel, W., & Fritz, R. (1991). Intravenous drug users and AIDS. *American Journal of Drug and Alcohol Abuse, 17,* 337–353.

Booth, R., Kwiatkowski, C., & Chitwood, D. (2000). Sex-related HIV risk behaviors: Differential risks among injection drug users, crack smokers, and injection drug users who smoke crack. *Drug and Alcohol Dependence, 58*(3), 219–226.

Booth, R., Kwiatkowski, C., & Stephens, R. (1998). Effectiveness of HIV/AIDS interventions on drug use and needle risk behaviors for out-of-treatment injection drug users. *Journal of Psychoactive Drugs, 30,* 269–278.

Boyd, C. J. (1993). The antecedents of women's crack cocaine abuse: Family substance abuse, sexual abuse, depression an illicit drug use. *Journal of Substance Abuse Treatment, 10*(5), 433–438.

Bux, D., Lamb, R., & Iguchi, M. (1995). Cocaine use and HIV risk behavior in methadone maintenance patients. *Drug and Alcohol Dependence, 37,* 29–35.

Carlson, R., Wang, J., Siegel, H., Falk, R., & Guo, J. (1994). An ethnographic approach to targeted sampling. *Human Organization, 53,* 279–295.

Chasnoff, I. (1988). Cocaine, pregnancy, and the neonate. *Women and Health, 15,* 23–25.

Chiasson, M., Stoneburner, R., Hildebrandt, D., Ewing, W., Telzak, E., & Jaffe, H. (1991). Heterosexual transmission of HIV-1 associated with the use of smokable freebase cocaine (crack). *AIDS, 5,* 1121–1126.

Chitwood, D., Inciardi, J., & McBride, D. (1991). *A community approach to AIDS intervention: Exploring the Miami outreach project for injecting drug users and other high risk groups.* Westport, CT: Greenwood Press.

Cohen, E., Navaline, H., & Metzger, D. (1994). High-risk behaviors for HIV: A comparison between crack-abusing and opioid-abusing African American women. *Journal of Psychoactive Drugs, 26,* 233–241.

Compton, W., Lamb, R., & Fletcher, B. (1995). Results of the NIDA treatment demonstration grants: cocaine workgroup: Characteristics of cocaine users and HIV risk behaviors. *Drug and Alcohol Dependence, 37,* 1–6.

Cottler, L. et al. (1998). Effectiveness of HIV risk reduction initiatives among out-of-treatment non-injection drug users. *Journal of Psychoactive Drugs, 30*(3), 279–290.

Deren, S., Tortu, S., & Davis, W. (1993). An AIDS risk reduction project with inner city women. In C. Squire (Ed.), *Women and AIDS* (pp. 73–89). London: Sage.

DesJarlais, D., Friedman, S., & Strug, D. (1986). AIDS and needle sharing within the IDU subculture. In D. Feldman & M. Johnson (Eds.), *The social dimensions of AIDS* (pp. 111–126). New York: Praeger.

DiClemente, R. J., & Wingood, G. M. (1995). A randomized controlled trial of an HIV sexual risk-reduction intervention for young African-American women. *Journal of the American Medical Association, 274,* 1271–1276.

Edlin, B., Irwin, K., Ferric, S., McCoy, B., Word, C., Serrano, Y., et al. (1994). Intersecting epidemics: Crack cocaine use and HIV infection among innercity young adults. *New England Journal of Medicine, 331,* 1422–1427.

El-Bassel, N., & Schilling, R. F. (1992). 15-month follow-up of women methadone patients taught skills to reduce heterosexual HIV transmission. *Public Health Reports, 107,* 500–504.

File, K. (1976). Sex roles and street roles. *International Journal of the Addictions, 11,* 263–268.

Fullilove, M., Fullilove, R., Bower, B., Haynes, R., & Gross, S. (1990). Black women and AIDS: Gender rules. *Journal of Sex Research, 27,* 47–64.

Geertz, C. (1973). *The interpretation of cultures: Selected essays.* New York: Basic Books.

Goldstein, P. (1979). *Prostitution and drug use.* Lexington, MA: Lexington Books.

Inciardi, J., Pottieger, D., & Lockwood, A. (1993). *Women and Crack Cocaine.* New York: Macmillan Press.

Jemmott, L. S., & Jemmott, J. B. (1992). Increasing condom-use intentions among sexually active black adolescent women. *Nursing Research, 41,* 273–279.

Johnson, B., et al. (1985). *Taking care of business: The economics of crime by heroin users.* Lexington, MA: Lexington Books.

Kane, S. (1991). HIV, heroin and heterosexual relations. *Social Science and Medicine, 32,* 1037–1050.

Kaplan, C., Korf, D., & Sterk, C. (1986). Temporal and social context of heroin-using populations: An illustration of the snowball sampling technique. *Journal of Nervous and Mental Diseases, 175,* 566–574.

Kearney, M., Murphy, S., & Rosenbaum, M. (1994). Mothering on crack cocaine: A grounded theory analysis. *Social Science and Medicine, 38,* 351–361.

King, V., Brooner, R., Bigelow, G., Schmidt, C., Flecht, L., & Gazaway, P. (1994). Condom use rates for specific sexual behaviors among opium users in treatment. *Drug and Alcohol Dependence, 35,* 231–238.

Latkin, C., Mandell, W., Vlahov, D., Oziemkowska, M., & Celentano, D. (1996). People and places: Behavioral settings and personal network characteristics as correlates of needle sharing. *Journal of Acquired Immune Deficiency Syndrome, 13,* 273–280.

Lieb, J., & Sterk-Elifson, C. (1995). Crack in the cradle: Reproductive decision making among crack cocaine users. *Journal of Contemporary Drug Problems, 12,* 687–706.

Mays, V., & Cochran, S. (1988). Interpretation of AIDS risk and risk-reduction activities by black and hispanic women. *Women Psychologist, 43,* 949–957.

McCoy, V., & Inciardi, J. (1993). Women and AIDS. *Women and Health, 20,* 69–86.

Neaigus, A., Friedman, S., Curtis, R., DesJarlais, D., Furst, R., Jose, B., et al. (1994). The relevance of drug injectors: Social networks and risk networks for understanding and preventing HIV infection. *Social Science and Medicine, 38,* 67–78.

Nyamathi, A., & Lewis, C. (1991). Coping of African-American women at risk for AIDS. *Women Health International, 1,* 53–62.

O'Leary, A. (1999). Preventing HIV infection in heterosexual women: What do we know? What must we learn? *Applied and Preventive Psychology, 8,* 257–263.

O'Leary, A., Goodhart, F., Jemmott, L., & Boccher-Lattimore, D. (1992). Predictors of safer sexual behavior on the college campus: A social cognitive theory analysis. *Journal of American College Health, 40,* 254–263.

Ouellet, L., Jimenez, W., & Johnson, W. (1991). Shooting galleries and HIV disease: Variations in places for injecting illicit drugs. *Crime and Delinquency, 36,* 64–85.

Prochaska, J., & DiClemente, C. (1983). Stages and processes of self-change of smoking. *Journal of Counseling and Clinical Psychology, 51,* 390–395.

Prochaska, J., DiClemente, C., & Norcross, J. (1992). In search of how people change. *American Psychologist, 47,* 1102–1114.

Ratner, M. (Ed.). (1993). *Crack pipe as a pimp.* Lexington, MA: Lexington Books.

Rosenbaum, M. (1981). *Women on heroin.* New Brunswick, NJ: Rutgers University Press.

Rosenstock, I. (1974). The health belief model and preventive health behavior. *Health Education Monograph, 2,* 328–335.

Rosenstock, I., Strecher, V., & Becker, M. (1988). Social Learning Theory and the Health Belief Model. *Health Education Quarterly, 15,* 175–183.

Siegel, H., Falk, R., Carlson, R., & Wang, J. (1995). Reducing HIV needle risk behavior among IDU in the Midwest. *AIDS Education and Prevention, 7,* 308–319.

Singer, M. (1991). Confronting the AIDS epidemic among IV drug users: Does ethnic culture matter? *AIDS Education and Prevention, 3,* 258–283.

Sterk, C. (1988). Cocaine and HIV Seropositivity. *The Lancet, 1,* 1052–1053.

Sterk C. (1999a). *Fast lives: Women who use crack cocaine.* Philadelphia: Temple University Press.

Sterk, C. (1999b). Building bridges: Community involvement in HIV and substance abuse research. *Drugs and Society, 14*(1–2), 107–121.

Sterk, C. (2000). *Tricking and tripping: Prostitution in the era of AIDS*. Putnam Valley, NY: Social Change Press.

Strauss, A., & Corbin, J. (1990). *Basics of qualitative research: Grounded theory procedures and techniques*. Newbury Park, CA: Sage.

Sutter, A. (1976). The world of the righteous dope fiend. *Issues in Criminology, 2*, 177–222.

Tashima, N., Crain, S., O'Reilly, K., & Sterk-Elifson, C. (1996). The community identification process: A discovery model. *Qualitative Health Research, 6*(1), 23–48.

Thomas, S., & Quinn, S. (1991). The Tuskeegee syphilis study, 1932–1972: Implications for HIV education and AIDS risk reduction programs in the black community. *American Journal of Public Health, 81*, 1498–1505.

Tortu, S., Beardsley, M., Deren, S., & Davis, W. (1994). The risk of HIV infection in a national sample of women with IDU partners. *American Journal of Public Health, 84*, 1243–1249.

Watters, J. K., & Biernacki, P. (1989). Targeted sampling: Options for the study of hidden populations. *Social Problems, 36*, 416–430.

Chapter 9

COMMUNITY INTERVENTION TRIALS: THEORETICAL AND METHODOLOGICAL CONSIDERATIONS

Ralph J. DiClemente, Richard A. Crosby, Catlainn Sionean, and David Holtgrave

OVERVIEW

Historically, individual- and group-level interventions have been designed to maximize interaction between intervenors and program recipients. The assumption underlying this approach, of course, is that these programs can be more intensive, more personalized, and can specifically target individuals' particular barriers to adopting and maintaining health-promoting behaviors. An alternate approach to individual- or group-level interventions involves targeting the community.

Community-level health-promotion programs are an extension of the more traditional intervention approaches. Given the magnitude of preventable chronic disease (particularly heart disease) and preventable infectious diseases (particularly infection with the human immunodeficiency virus and sexually transmitted diseases), expanding program delivery to the community level amplifies the odds that substantial numbers of people will ultimately be exposed to the intervention and may adopt health protective behaviors.

One important advantage of delivering programs at the community level is that reaching a broad proportion of the community may result in changing existing community norms so that they are more supportive of health-protection behaviors. In turn, these new norms may prompt continued diffusion of health-protective behaviors, reaching beyond individuals directly exposed to the intervention (Farquhar, 1978). Community-level intervention strategies may also be more effective than individual- or group-level intervention strategies because they integrate multiple levels of influence. For example, community-level intervention strategies may involve institutional, organizational, community, and policy influences designed to amplify the adoption and maintenance of health promoting behaviors as well as factors designed to affect intrapersonal and interpersonal influences on health behavior (Emmons, 2000; McLeroy, Bibeau, Steckler, & Glanz, 1988).

Rationale for Community-Level Interventions

There has been a marked change in the etiology of disease in the United States. Early in the twentieth century, disease was mainly attributable to infectious pathogens. However, by midcentury a significant trend emerged that identified chronic diseases as the primary cause of morbidity and mortality. Since this epidemiological transition from infectious to chronic disease, health and illness have been perceived largely as a function of behavior. This *individualistic perspective* has dominated the field of health promotion and disease prevention for the past 50 years (McLeroy et al., 1988).

In recent years, a shift has occurred from focusing on the individual to focusing on the community. The definition of *community* varies considerably in the literature. Traditionally, it refers to groups of people with shared values and institutions. Thus, *community* necessarily includes social meaning and organizational structures. Alternatively, in much research, *community* is often operationalized as groups of individuals with a shared geographic location.

The roots of community-level interventions to enhance health-protecting behaviors lie in the history of epidemiology. This field began to emerge in the seventeenth century, with the observation that the burden of disease and death disproportionately affects impoverished groups (Susser & Susser, 1996). By the nineteenth century, rapidly accelerating industrialization magnified existing disparities between social classes. This had the effect of spurring documentation of the distribution of disease in populations. As specific organisms had yet to be observed, the prevailing theory of disease etiology was miasma (impure water, air, etc.). Thus, disease prevention efforts were directed toward populations and utilized changes in the environment, such as improved sanitation and sewage removal.

Beginning in the mid-nineteenth century, epidemiologists began to suspect that microorganisms could cause disease. As discussed in chapter 1, in 1854, John Snow turned off the Broad Street pump, in culmination of his research demonstrating that the water from one particular supplier was related to high rates of cholera. Scientific advances led to the discovery of microorganisms as causes of disease; thus began the era of infectious disease epidemiology. The prevailing theory guiding disease prevention in this era was germ theory. Thus, attempts to prevent disease involved the prevention of transmission of infectious agents, through means such as vaccination and quarantine (Susser & Susser, 1996).

By the mid-twentieth century, in developed nations, chronic diseases—notably coronary heart disease and lung cancer—replaced infectious diseases as the primary causes of mortality, prompting a need for a new theoretical model of disease causation (Cassel, 1964). The now familiar case-control study design was used to determine risk factors, or characteristics of individuals with disease relative to those without disease. More powerful predictive designs also began to be utilized, namely, the cohort study. In this design, researchers sought to identify increased risk for developing particular diseases among those with defined characteristics relative to those without these characteristics (i.e., relative risk). Concurrently, a new field, health promotion, emerged, informed largely by cognitive psychology, (Breslow, 1999). As a result, the primary theory of etiology, and hence the prevailing strategy for disease prevention, came to focus increasingly on the individual.

Individual-level strategies for disease prevention seek to identify individuals at high risk for developing particular diseases based on their risk behaviors or characteristics. This strategy is based on a clinical model. That is, it seeks to identify and change causes of individual cases of disease, for instance, through physicians' screening their patients for risk factors. Once high-risk individuals are identified, interventions informed by this perspective attempt to reduce the risk of developing disease primarily through modifying the risk behaviors (e.g., lifestyle factors such as smoking and diet) associated with the particular disease. Psychological theories widely applied to health behavior have included the theory of reasoned action (Ajzen & Fishbein, 1980), social cognitive theory (Bandura, 1977, 1997), and transtheoretical model of behavior change (DiClemente & Prochaska, 1998). Given the common use of these and other psychology-based theories, interventions have been designed to address important proximal antecedents to risk behaviors such as knowledge, attitudes, beliefs, motivation, peer norms, risk reduction, self-efficacy, and skill acquisition. Such interventions have demonstrated evidence of effectiveness in reducing or delaying the adoption of disease-associated risk behaviors, such as smoking (Prochaska, DiClemente, Velicer, & Rossi, 1993), substance use, and sexual risk behaviors (Centers for Disease Control and Prevention [CDC], 1999a).

Although the individual approach has been successful, it has several disadvantages (Rose, 1985, 1992). First, screening to identify individuals at high risk can be both costly and pragmatically difficult. Many disease processes of greatest concern, such as arteriosclerosis, begin early in life; thus, screening would have to be implemented early and repeated at regular intervals. In addition, participation in screening programs is often greatest among those individuals who are at lower risk for disease (i.e., the "worried well"). Thus, screening programs may fail to identify many individuals who are at risk.

Second, even with screening programs for diseases that are prevalent in a population, the ability to predict which individuals will develop future disease is typically weak. Prediction is weak because the majority of cases may be comprised of individuals at low to moderate risk, rather than those few individuals identified as high-risk.

Finally, and most important, the behaviors often targeted for change by individual-level interventions (e.g., smoking, dietary habits, physical activity, and unprotected sexual activity) are inherently social and are therefore influenced by forces external to individuals, such as prevailing social norms, public policy, and factors inherent in the physical environment. Thus, individual-level intervention strategies, though pragmatic and yielding modest effects, may not be optimally efficacious for enhancing the adoption of health-promoting behaviors. In addition, and equally important from a public health perspective, individual-level intervention strategies may be insufficient to sustain newly adopted health behaviors over prolonged periods of time, particularly in the context of pervasive social pressures that promote or reinforce risk behavior.

In sum, individual-level approaches to health promotion are often palliative and temporary because they are not capable of reaching large segments of the at-risk population. Thus, though the approach may benefit small numbers of recipients, large numbers of people are at-risk but never identified; at-risk and identified but do not participate in the program; or not at-risk but—perhaps in the absence of exposure to a program—subsequently move into the at-risk population.

Nature of Community-Level Interventions

The metaphor of pulling people who are drowning from a river is useful in comparing individual-level strategies to community-level strategies. The individual-level strategy has been referred to as a "downstream" approach because it focuses interventions on pulling drowning individuals from the river's currents (i.e., individuals who already have risk factors associated with disease occurrence). Alternatively, the community-level strategy can be conceptualized as an upstream approach because it looks "upstream" to see what is pushing individuals into the river in the first place (Zola, quoted in McKinlay, 1974). Thus, the community-level approach focuses predominantly on keeping people from falling in the river (i.e., acquiring risk factors associated with disease occurrence). A variant on the community-level approach is to target high-risk communities and attempt to reduce risk behaviors.

To focus on those at highest risk is only a temporary solution, because even if an intervention successfully motivates individuals to change their high-risk behaviors, other individuals are constantly entering the high-risk population to replace them. Thus, individual-based interventions may have only limited effects because they do not change the distribution of risk behavior in the population as a whole. Illustrative of this conceptualization is a quote from the Multiple Risk Factor Intervention Trial (MRFIT):

> [E]very time we helped a man in [MRFIT] to stop smoking, on that day, probably one to two children in a schoolyard somewhere are taking their first tentative puffs on a cigarette for the first time. So, even when we do help high-risk people to lower their risk, we do nothing to change the distribution of disease in the population because, in one-to-one programs . . . we do nothing to influence forces in society that caused the problem in the first place. (Syme, 1996, p. 463)

The community-level approach to disease prevention is based not on a medical model but on a public health model. That is, it seeks to change not simply individuals or groups of individuals but the distribution of disease in the population as a whole. To change the average level of risk factors and disease prevalence, the community-level approach looks upstream to determine which characteristics of the community may influence the health status of the community as a whole (prevalence) as well as those that directly or indirectly influence individual risk.

A substantial body of research indicates that characteristics of communities may have an important influence on health outcomes and individual risk behaviors (Cohen, Spear, et al., 2000; Robert, 1998). Ecological studies have documented associations between community-level social and economic conditions and a variety of health outcomes (Acevedo-Garcia, 2001; Cohen, Spear, et al., 2000; Friedman, Perlis, & DeJarlais, 2001; Kaplan, Pamuk, Lynch, Cohen, & Balfour, 1996; Lynch et al., 1998). Moreover, community characteristics are associated directly and indirectly with individuals' risks for poor health outcomes, even after controlling for the effects of individual characteristics (Diez-Roux et al., 1997; O'Campo, Xue, Wang, & Caughy, 1997).

One particularly important determinant of health behaviors across members of a given community may be the level of social capital in the community. As noted by Putnam, the term "social capital" has been redefined numerous times (Putnam, 2000). Although there is a lack of consensus with respect to the definition of social capital, there is an emerging consensus that social capital is comprised of a small set of central core factors that include trust, reciprocity, and cooperation among members of a social network that aims to achieve common goals. The term includes supportive interactions within and among families, neighborhoods, and entire communities (Putnam, 2000). For example, recent studies suggest that one potentially important community-level predictor of sexual risk behavior among adolescents may be their affiliation with organized social groups (Crosby, DiClemente, Wingood, Harrington, Davies, Hook, et al., 2002; Crosby, DiClemente, Wingood, Harrington, Davies, & Malow, 2002; Ramirez-Valles, Zimmerman, & Newcomb, 1998; Schinke, Orlandi, & Cole, 1992). In addition, social capital has been related to numerous public health measures such as child welfare, violent behavior, mortality, and health status (Kawachi, Kennedy, & Glass, 1999; Kawachi, Kennedy, Lochner, & Prothrow-Stith, 1997; Kreuter & Lezin, 2002; Putnam, 2000). Generally, higher levels of social capital are associated with more favorable health indices. For example, a recent study found that higher social capital was associated with fewer deficits in emotional, behavioral, and developmental functioning among preschool children (Runyan et al., 1998). Greater levels of social capital, assessed by state, have also been significantly associated with lower state-level rates of AIDS, gonorrhea, and syphilis among adolescents and adults (Holtgrave, Crosby, DiClemente, Wingood, & Gayle, 2002). These studies collectively suggest that interventions designed to enhance community social capital may be a valuable strategy for promoting health.

In sum, community-level interventions are designed to promote widespread behavior change by utilizing naturally occurring channels of influence (e.g., social and friendship networks) and social institutions (e.g., media, organized religion), while simultaneously providing supportive environmental structures that encourage the adoption and maintenance of health-protective behaviors.

Purpose of Community-Level Interventions

The primary purpose of population-based strategies (i.e., community-level interventions) to disease prevention is to shift downward the mean level of risk factors in a given population. As demonstrated in Figure 9.1, this reduction in mean risk may effectively reduce the bell portion of the curve, resulting in a shift that moves people from high risk to moderate risk or from moderate risk to low risk (Rose, 1985, 1992).

Community-level approaches are based on the concept of population-attributable risk, that is, the amount of disease in a given population attributable to a specified level of exposure (Hennekens & Buring, 1987). Population-attributable risk is typically greatest in the central part of a disease distribution (i.e., in the bell part of a normal curve). Thus, the majority of the cases may be observed among individuals with only moderate levels of risk factors (e.g., heart disease, diabetes, and many types of malignancies). The community-level approach therefore seeks to identify and alter the underlying forces within communities that make the disease so prevalent in a given population. That is, rather than attempt to identify characteristics of individuals that place them at risk for a particular disease, the community-level approach identifies socioenvironmental factors that are likely to (a) predispose individuals to the adoption of risk behavior; (b) prevent individuals from adopting protective behavior; or (c) lead directly to increased risk for disease, regardless of individuals' risk behaviors (e.g., environmental toxins) (Link & Phelan, 1995).

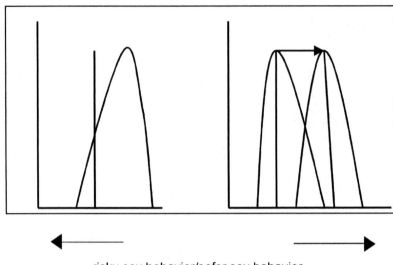

risky sex behavior/safer sex behavior

Individual-level interventions   Community-level interventions
                                       ("shift the curve")

FIGURE 9.1 Schematic depiction of community-level intervention shifting the mean level of HIV-associated risk factors in a downward direction.

STRUCTURE OF COMMUNITY-LEVEL INTERVENTIONS

Distinguishing Aspects

As previously described, interventions may attempt to promote behavior change at the individual level or at the larger community level. In addition, interventions may be implemented through a variety of different venues, ranging from families to worksites and finally to communities. It is important to distinguish between *community-based* and *community-level* interventions. Many community interventions are delivered in community settings, such as schools, worksites, and so forth, and may address important features of the community. However, such an intervention may still be individually based if it is designed to change (exclusively) the behavior of the individuals who participate in the intervention. Community-level interventions seek to alter the physical or social environmental characteristics of communities. In essence then, the hallmark of community-level approaches is their emphasis on changing physical or social conditions (Sweat & Denison, 1995). Some distinguishing characteristics of community-level approaches include improving *availability,* improving *physical resources,* and communicating through *community events and media channels* (Cohen, Scribner, & Farley, 2000).

Availability. Access to health-promoting or health-compromising products or services can change behavior without influencing individuals' attitudes. Accessibility to harmful products such as tobacco and alcohol may be reduced by limiting locations and times for sales or by increasing prices. Programs and policies may also be used to increase access to harm reduction products, for example, needle exchange and condom distribution programs. Readily available products (e.g., nutritious foods, exercise facilities) may also be an objective of the intervention program.

Physical Resources. Deteriorating environments may create conditions that lead to health-risk behaviors such as drug use and prostitution. In addition, these environments may indicate community members' tacit approval for engaging in risky behaviors such as substance abuse and violence. Change in the physical environment may also be a direct route to reducing the incidence of infectious diseases (Garrett, 1994).

Community Events and Media Channels. These channels have the capacity to reduce risks for a large numbers of people because the people are passively exposed to the intervention. As health behaviors are adopted by progressively larger proportions of a community, the increased social acceptability of these behaviors may help promote adoption of health behaviors and, subsequently, reinforce maintenance of health behaviors among those initially unexposed to the intervention through diffusion effects (Rogers, 1995).

Despite the benefits of the community-level approach, it does have some disadvantages, for instance, the "prevention paradox." That is, community-level interventions are not tailored to individuals and therefore many individuals may not readily perceive the intrinsic value of the intervention. As a consequence, community-level interventions typically offer little immediate benefit to some individuals because they may not attend to the messages. In addition, many will not benefit because they are not at risk and thus would be unlikely to develop the disease or condition in question.

Recent theoretical and statistical advances have prompted the emergence of a new class of intervention designed to capitalize on the strengths of both the individual and community-level approaches. These multilevel interventions utilize components of various social contexts in which individuals are embedded (worksite, schools, families). Such interventions have the potential to work synergistically, mutually reinforcing and facilitating changes made by individuals. Indeed, multilevel interventions have been implemented and have shown promising results in areas such as alcohol and tobacco use.

The use of community-level interventions, particularly multilevel interventions in which individuals are also targeted for change, necessarily requires careful attention to design and analytical plans. In the following section, several important methodological concerns of community-level interventions are described.

Design and Analytic Issues

The design of community-level interventions is intimately linked to a host of analytic issues; thus, design and analysis should be planned concurrently. For example, a primary feature of community intervention trials is that the unit of observation is typically the individual, but the unit of randomization and analysis is usually the community. However, many community-level intervention trials do not randomly assign communities to treatment conditions because doing so would present insurmountable practical and political barriers, thus giving rise to quasi-experimental research designs (i.e., designs that lack randomization). However, quasi-experimental designs are not necessarily undesirable. Although they lack the internal validity provided by experimental designs, they may be a better approximation of the real world and therefore have greater external validity.

Community-level trials are unique in that they typically involve few units of analysis, because the unit of analysis is usually the community rather than the individual. This creates multiple problems. For example, Murray (1998) noted that even with random assignment of communities in community-level trials, randomization may not always be effective. In trials involving small numbers of communities (e.g., Stanford, Pawtucket, and Minnesota-based heart health programs) randomization is unlikely to achieve its intended purpose, i.e., symmetric distribution of potential bias across intervention and control communities. Without symmetrical distribution of potential bias, systematic error can easily distort study findings.

The few units of analysis in community-level interventions also give rise to low statistical power. Several solutions have been suggested to remedy problems associated with low statistical power. For example, Murray (1998) emphasized measurement of all possible sources of variance, assuring that all statistical assumptions are met, and designing the study to focus on a single, primary, endpoint. An additional solution is to analyze the unit of observation (i.e., individuals) and statistically control for similarities with the unit of randomization (i.e., account for the intraclass correlation often observed within clusters such as communities).

Despite methods of compensating for low statistical power, the majority of community-level interventions have been underpowered, resulting in only weak evidence, at best, supporting their effectiveness (Fishbein, 1996). Fishbein pointed out that community-level programs often lack power to detect even medium effect sizes, let alone small effect sizes. Yet small effect sizes in community-level interventions may be very meaningful at the population level. Furthermore, Fishbein also noted that power could be enhanced by precisely defining the behavioral endpoint of the community-level intervention and defining/clarifying the outcome measure with precision.

Koepsell, Diehr, Cheadle, and Kristal (1995) pointed out that loss of statistical power in community-level interventions commonly results from matching communities on variables that are not strongly correlated to the outcome measures. Accordingly, they advocated matching communities based on careful assessments of associations between community characteristics and trial endpoints. This process requires time and resources to conduct thorough preliminary analyses of the communities. Although the practice advocated by Koepsell and colleagues can result in increased statistical power, this practice is not usually included in the design of community-level interventions.

Another unique aspect of community-level interventions is the delivery of the programs to an entire target population. Similarity of persons within a target population facilitates intervention design and delivery. However, it also poses analytic problems. Observations of members in the same target population tend to be correlated. To avoid potential bias in study conclusions, this correlation within communities must be accounted for statistically (Murray, 1995). Conversely, using the community as the unit of analysis avoids this potential bias entirely.

Studies of community-level interventions typically use either nested cross-sectional, nested cohort, or a combination of the two designs. Much like cohort studies commonly used in epidemiologic research, nested cohort studies prospectively follow groups of people who are selected only from defined communities. Alternatively, nested cross-sectional studies require successive waves of surveys administered to random samples of community members. One problem with this approach is that the time of year when the survey is administered must be common across each community (Murray, 1995). In addition, measures should be taken to avoid an interactive effect between the community and the person administering the survey (Murray, 1998). In the context of nested cohort designs, a common problem is high attrition rates.

An additional issue with community-level interventions is community selection. Community selection should be based on several criteria, including ample distance (including nonoverlapping media markets) between selected communities to avoid contamination effects. If communities will be randomized, then all communities involved must first express willingness to be assigned to the experimental condition. Clearly, the process of defining community willingness is complex (chapter 1). At this stage, it is important to work with communities to secure their involvement, identify key decision-makers, and obtain their support for the trial.

When communities are matched, care should be taken to assert that they do not differ with respect to potential sociodemographic confounders, for example, race, age, income, and education. When differences between matched communities are discovered, they should be controlled for statistically. A particularly important confounding variable that should be avoided is the existence of similar programs in either the intervention or comparison communities. Similar programs in the comparison communities create a bias toward a null finding, whereas similar programs in the intervention communities create a bias toward the research hypothesis. Because controlling the existence of similar programs is not feasible or desirable, it is important to assess and understand their potential contribution toward study bias.

A variety of design and analytic approaches have been applied to community-level interventions, and many of these are reviewed in the following sections.

The AIDS Community Demonstration Projects

Design. One of the most recent large-scale community-level intervention trials was conducted by the Centers for Disease Control and Prevention (CDC, 1999b). The study was a nested cross-sectional design, that is, repeated cross-sectional surveys were conducted within both the intervention and comparison communities during the course of the project. Table 9.1 schematically describes the trial design.

Communities were defined by specific at-risk populations (e.g., commercial sex workers and non-gay-identified men who have sex with men) within defined geographic boundaries. Communities were matched by pairs, according to selected sociodemographic criteria. Unfortunately, random assignment to condition was only possible in 1 of 5 community pairs, making the design quasi-experimental.

Analysis. Baseline data was collected by two survey waves. Eight successive survey waves followed over the course of a 32-month intervention. The intervention had three components: verbal and written prevention messages delivered by community members; small media campaigns; and availability of condoms and bleach kits. Exposure to the intervention was defined as self-reported contact with any one of these intervention components. The trial endpoint was defined as

TABLE 9.1 Schematic of the Study Design for the AIDS Community Demonstration Projects

| Procedure | Matched Intervention-Comparison Communities | | | | |
	Pair 1	Pair 2	Pair 3	Pair 4	Pair 5
Baseline survey	X/X	X/X	X/X	X/X	X/X
Baseline survey	X/X	X/X	X/X	X/X	X/X
Begin 32-month intervention	X/O	X/O	X/O	X/O	X/O
Repeat surveys at 7 intervals	X/X	X/X	X/X	X/X	X/X
End 32-month intervention	X/O	X/O	X/O	X/O	X/O
Final survey	X/X	X/X	X/X	X/X	X/X

Note: X/X = both communities in the pair; X/O = only the designated intervention community in the pair progress along the stages of change (SOC) continuum (Prochaska et al., 1993).

Regression techniques were used to (a) assess adjusted mean scores for SOC within each of the 10 communities, and (b) assess change in mean community-level SOC scores over time. Individual-level analyses were also conducted to determine adjusted associations between exposure to the intervention and the trial endpoints.

Community-Level HIV Prevention Programs for Women

Design. A recent community-level HIV prevention project, based largely on methods used in the CDC Demonstration Projects, was conducted for communities of low-income women (Lauby, Smith, Stark, Person, & Adams, 2000). The Prevention of HIV in Women and Infants Demonstration Project (WIDP) used a nested cross-sectional design to evaluate the impact of a 2-year community-level intervention delivered in four locations. After identification of the intervention communities, matched comparison communities were selected. Although annual cross-sectional surveys were conducted over a 4-year period, only the baseline and the last postintervention survey wave were used to evaluate program effectiveness.

Sikkema and colleagues (2000) also conducted and evaluated a community-level HIV prevention program for women. The project involved a large number of communities across five geographically diverse cities in the United States. Eighteen communities of women living in low-income housing were matched into nine pairs and surveyed at baseline. Each matched pair was randomly assigned to the intervention or control condition, with one exception: one community was assigned to the intervention condition but did not have space available for a portion of the planned intervention. The intervention lasted 1 year. Although the follow-up survey was also cross-sectional, sufficient numbers of women in each community were resurveyed to conduct a nested cohort analysis. This procedure, combined with the large number of communities involved, resulted in substantially more statistical power than the study reported by Lauby and colleagues (2000).

Analysis. In the study reported by Lauby and colleagues (2000), controlled analyses compared the average difference in change scores between the four intervention and four comparison communities. This same analysis was repeated using only data for women in the intervention communities who reported any exposure to the intervention (64%) and for those in the comparison communities reporting no exposure to the intervention (77%).

However, Sikkema and colleagues (2000) used a technique based on the generalized linear model (GLM) to analyze their cohort data. This family of models, like others used in community-level interventions, seeks to control for all possible sources of variance in order to optimize the chances of finding a significant interaction between study condition and time. Using GLM partitions variance by both the individual and group affiliation. Thus, it is possible to observe changes within an individual across time, as well as between groups (i.e., the intervention versus a comparison group) over time. An effective intervention would yield a group-by-time interaction showing that participants randomized to the intervention group demonstrated greater improvement relative to the comparison group over time. Like the approach used by Lauby and colleagues (2000), Sikkema and colleagues also conducted analyses adjusted for exposure to the intervention; however, the technique they used was somewhat different. About three quarters of the cohort residing in communities receiving the intervention reported attending at least two of the risk-reduction workshops that were offered as part of the overall intervention program. These women were compared to the entire cohort of women residing in the comparison community.

Pawtucket Heart Health Program

The Pawtucket Heart Health Program (PHHP) used a research design based on only a single intervention and a single comparison community (Carleton, Lasater, Assaf, Feldman, & McKinlay, 1995). The unique challenges inherent in such a restricted design were described by Murray (1998) and included inflated probabilities of systematic bias due to local history, differential maturation, and contamination. The PHHP supplemented the nested cross-sectional design with a nested cohort design.

Minnesota Heart Health Program

Like the PHHP, the Minnesota Heart Health Program (MHHP) also used a nested cohort design to supplement a nested cross-sectional design (Luepker et al., 1994). Unlike the PHHP, the MHHP used three matched pairs of communities. The intervention was initiated in a lagged fashion (that is, starting dates were staggered) across the three intervention cities, allowing for several baseline data collection points (thus allowing for improved precision in statistical analyses). Cohort surveys were conducted 2 years after the starting the intervention for one half of the cohort members, and 4 years after starting for the remaining half of the cohort.

A Community-Level HIV Prevention Program for Gay Men

Design.   Kelly and colleagues (1997) selected 16 small U.S. cities for a two-phase project; however, the project was not completed in eight of the cities that comprised phase two of the project. Although the project was implemented in all 16 cities, practical issues led to failure of the study and inability to implement phase two appropriately. The published trial results focused on eight cities, two in each of four states, which were randomized to a control or intervention condition by state. Paired cities were geographically isolated from each other, preventing problems with site contamination.

At least five nested cross-sectional surveys of men attending one of several gay bars were conducted 2 months before the intervention and 12 months after the intervention. Surveys were conducted during 3 consecutive nights and excluded men in long-term monogamous relationships. If the men completed more than one survey, data analysis was based only on the first survey completed.

The intervention was also conducted in gay bars. Gay bars in intervention cities displayed and distributed printed HIV prevention messages. In addition, these bars became venues for dissemination of prevention messages delivered by trained peer leaders (peer opinion leader model). In the control cities, only the printed HIV prevention messages were utilized in the gay bars.

Analysis.   City-level and individual-level analyses were conducted. Dependent measures were assessed by self-report, using a recall period of 6 months. These included frequency of unprotected anal sex, the proportion of those surveyed reporting any unprotected anal sex, the percent of condom use during anal sex, and the number of anal sex partners. To validate the self-reported measures, the adjusted percent of free condoms taken from bars was also assessed. Regression techniques were used to detect condition by time interactions for the city-level outcome data.

Two similar studies have been conducted. Kelly and colleagues (1992) assessed the effects of a similar intervention using peer leaders. Similar to Kelly (1997), this study found reductions in unprotected anal sex and increases in condom-protected anal sex among gay men attending bars. This study took place in three small cities; however, each city received the intervention. The experiment was controlled by using a sequential stepwise lagged design; that is, the intervention was introduced by turn in each of the three cities with the second and third cities serving as controls for the city preceding them. This procedure involved five cross-sectional survey waves, with the intervention being provided to city one after wave two; to city two after wave three; and to city three after wave four (Table 9.2). Thus, the design was capable of detecting intervention effects as the interventions were sequentially administered. Because all three cities received the intervention, randomization was not necessary.

Another study similar to the one reported by Kelly and colleagues (1997) was reported by Kegeles, Hayes, and Coates (1996): The Mpowerment Project. The unit of analysis was the individual, and the unit of randomization was the community. Unlike the 1997 study by Kelly and colleagues, the Mpowerment Project used a nested cohort design. In this design, a sample of gay men from the intervention community and the comparison community were recruited separately

TABLE 9.2 Schematic of the Sequential Stepwise Lagged Design Used by Kelly and Colleagues

Procedure	City		
	City 1	City 2	City 3
Baseline survey	X	X	X
Baseline survey	X	X	X
Intervention	X		
Follow-up survey	X	X	X
Intervention		X	
Follow-up survey	X	X	X
Intervention			X
Follow-up survey	X	X	X

Note: X = administration of survey/intervention
Three months elapsed between administration periods, and the period of recall for dependent measures was 2 months.

and prior to starting the intervention program. The intervention lasted 8 months. Four months after concluding the intervention members of each cohort were asked to complete follow-up surveys. Retention was 65% in the intervention community and 88% in the comparison community.

Project COMMIT: An Anti-Smoking Program

Design. The Community Intervention Trial for Smoking Cessation (COMMIT) was a 4-year intervention conducted in randomly assigned cities within 11 matched city-pairs. The design was a combination of nested cross-sectional surveys and nested cohort surveys. Unlike other projects targeting multiple risk factors, COMMIT was designed specifically to encourage people to quit smoking, particularly heavy smokers. All surveys were conducted by telephone. Although cohort members were contacted annually by phone, only data from the prevalence survey conducted after conclusion of the intervention were used to test the primary study hypothesis. A portion of the cohort (80%) was randomly selected for follow-up relative to rates of smoking cessation. The remaining 20% provided a process evaluation of the intervention (e.g., awareness of, and participation in, program activities, recognition of smoking as a public health issue, and change in the social acceptability of smoking).

Analysis. Only community-level analyses were conducted. The mean of all possible pair-wise community differences in the dichotomous outcome was used to establish a significance level for hypothesis testing (known as a permutation test). One-sided permutation tests and corresponding 90% confidence intervals were used to test the study hypothesis. Two different procedures were used to account for missing data, with each yielding similar results. In addition, associations between quitting and level of intervention exposure were quantified, and logistic regression was used to adjust for possible confounders that were included in the regression models as covariates. This analytic procedure as applied in COMMIT has been advocated and described as being robust in publications by Green (1997), Green and colleagues (1995), and Koepsell and colleagues (1995).

EFFECTIVENESS OF COMMUNITY-LEVEL INTERVENTIONS

General Observations

Generally speaking, individual-level intervention trials are tightly controlled, methodologically rigorous studies designed to evaluate whether
a given intervention is efficacious in reducing health risk behaviors
(e.g., smoking). This level of rigor, however, is not a practical objective
in the context of community-level trials. Nonetheless, there is an advantage to this lack of rigor in that the study conditions are more representative of a real-world experience. Thus, findings from community-level
trials are much more likely than those from individual-level trials to
represent the true effect on the target population. It is important to note
that even small effects observed from community-level interventions
can translate into clinically significant improvements for the community
as a whole.

The following discussion of effectiveness for various community-
level trials (trials already presented in this chapter) is organized by
interventions targeting multiple risk behaviors versus those targeting
single risk behaviors. As might be expected, successful outcomes are
more common with the latter than with the former.

Effectiveness of Projects Targeting Multiple Risk Behaviors

The AIDS Community Demonstration Projects (ACDP) produced some
promising indicators that community-level interventions can reduce the
frequency of various HIV-risk behaviors within an entire population.
Using the community as the level of analysis, change in mean stage-
of-change (SOC) scores did not vary by assignment of community to
condition in regards to a key behavioral objective (use of bleach kits).
However, using the individual as the level analyses indicated that those
exposed to the intervention had higher SOC scores than those not
exposed.

At the final survey wave, increases in mean SOC scores for condom
use with a main partner were greater for the intervention as opposed
to the comparison communities. Increases in mean SOC community
scores for condom use with non-main partners were greater for intervention as opposed to comparison communities. Individual-level analy-

ses showed those exposed to the intervention had higher SOC scores for condom use with main and non-main partners. Condom carrying was more common in intervention communities, at both the community and individual level.

Of note, although the ACDP did not produce significant *community-level* findings for the use of bleach kits, Rietmeijer and colleagues (1996) found increased use of bleach kits among members of an intervention community in contrast to a comparison community using a nested cross-sectional design.

The 18-city community-level HIV prevention program for women reported by Sikkema and colleagues (2000) showed some promising results. The percent of women reporting any unprotected sex in the past two months declined from 50% to 38% among women in the intervention communities. Likewise, women living in intervention communities reported more frequent use of condoms.

Community-level intervention targeting gay men living in small cities and at risk of HIV have also shown some promising results (Kegeles et al., 1996; Kelly et al., 1992, 1997). For example, in the multiple-city study reported by Kelly and colleagues (1997), significant reductions in unprotected anal sex and increases in condom-protected anal sex were observed for the intervention cities as compared to the control cities. Differences were not found for the number of sexual partners. Of importance, significantly more condoms were distributed in the intervention cities, supporting the validity of the self-reported outcome data.

Findings reported by Kelly and colleagues (1992) and Kegeles and colleagues (1996) add to the weight of evidence that community-level approaches may be an effective method of reducing HIV risk among gay men attending gay bars on a regular basis. In each study significant declines in unprotected anal sex were observed among members of the intervention community, but not among members of the comparison community. Studies did not show significant decreases in the number of sexual partners.

Three large-scale intervention trials have been conducted to determine if community-level interventions can reduce severity of assessed risk factors for heart disease and reduce actual heart disease morbidity and mortality. The Stanford Five-City Project produced mixed findings (see chapter 10). As opposed to people surveyed in comparison cities, those interviewed or assessed in the intervention cities maintained improvements in blood pressure. In addition, individuals in the intervention cities maintained or demonstrated a decrease in coronary-heart-disease-related morbidity and mortality after the intervention, whereas those in the comparison cities leveled out or experienced increased levels of coronary-heart-disease-related morbidity and mortality. Compared to the intervention condition, individuals in the comparison cities experienced greater postintervention gain in CHD-prevention knowledge, greater postintervention decline in prevalence of smoking, and greater declines in body mass index (Fortmann et al., 1995; Winkleby, Taylor, Jatulis, & Fortmann, 1996).

Unfortunately, findings from the PHHP provided only weak evidence of an intervention effect. Null findings may be attributable to the low statistical power inherent in community-level analyses, particularly when only one community receives the intervention (Murray, 1998). Findings from the Minnesota Heart Health Program also failed to observe an intervention effect (Luepker et al., 1994).

Effectiveness of Projects Targeting Single Behaviors

Project COMMIT (COMMIT Research Group, 1995a, 1995b) showed that a community-level intervention could produce significant declines in the number of community members who originally reported light to moderate cigarette use. These findings were consistent between the cross-sectional data and the cohort data. Extended analyses revealed a correlation between level of exposure to the intervention activities and quitting cigarette use. However, the intervention did not impact those who originally reported heavy use of cigarettes.

The Prevention of HIV in Women and Infants Demonstration Project (WIDP) examined change in condom use behaviors. Evaluation of WIDP indicated that women in the intervention communities were more likely than women in comparison communities to report increased effort to persuade their main partners to use condoms. In addition, women in the intervention communities were more likely to report talking about condom use with their main partners. A marginal intervention effect was observed indicating that women in the intervention communities were more likely to report any use of condoms. Intervention effects on condom use for women in relationships with casual partners were not found. Subgroup analyses that included women exposed in the intervention communities and not inadvertently exposed in the comparison communities (no contamination) revealed that women in the intervention communities were more likely than those in the comparison communities to increase their efforts to persuade casual partners to use condoms.

Caveats to Interpreting Findings From Community
Intervention Trials

Community-level designs and their respective analytic methods may overrepresent or underrepresent effectiveness of the intervention. Thus, several factors should be considered after the analyses show either significant or nonsignificant results. Some of the more important factors follow:

1.   In nested cohort designs, findings may be biased by differences between the cohort and the community represented by the cohort. This may be particularly likely when cohort participation rates are low and attrition rates are high, creating a bias. Consequently, findings may not be representative of the communities (Blumenthal, Sung, Williams, Liff, & Coates, 1995).

2.   Assessed endpoints in community-level trials may underrepresent the effectiveness of the intervention. Endpoints such as blood pressure, body mass index, and cardiovascular morbidity and mortality may not capture the full range of behavior change in a population. Each of these endpoints is influenced by genetic factors and historical factors that predispose to CHD and may not be amenable to change. Thus, null findings may not represent lack of behavior change. Utilizing changes in risk behaviors (i.e., diet, smoking) rather than strictly relying on changes in biological outcomes (i.e., CHD) may better reflect intervention effectiveness (Fishbein, 1996).

Efficient indicators of program success may be as simple as the amount of fresh fruits and vegetables purchased in a community that is receiving a nutrition enhancement program, the number of condoms purchased in a community that is receiving an HIV prevention program, or the number of restaurants developing nonsmoking policies in a community that is receiving a tobacco use prevention program (Koepsell et al., 1995).

3.   Community-level interventions that designate the individual as the unit of analysis may thereby overrepresent their findings. A basic statistical principle is that the unit of randomization is usually the unit of analysis. Community-level intervention trials should be designed with enough power to detect even small effect sizes using the community as the unit of analysis. Power is increased by (a) adding more communities, (b) ensuring similarity across communities, (c) designing effective intervention strategies tailored to very

specific and achievable endpoints, and (d) using one-tailed significance tests (a procedure commonly practiced in community-level
analysis).

SUMMARY

Community-level health promotion programs hold great promise for
significantly impacting morbidity and mortality. However, though these
interventions may be more efficacious and cost-effective relative to
traditional individual-level intervention strategies, a number of thorny
methodological hurdles must be surmounted to evaluate these programs. There is an overriding need for methodological rigor to ade-
quately evaluate community-level programs. Thus, though the potential
for community-level health promotion interventions is substantial, we
must countenance the methodological challenges to demonstrate that
community-level programs can positively impact the adoption and maintenance of health-protective behaviors, attitudes, norms, and beliefs.
Only with a coordinated and systematic research agenda can we hope
to isolate and quantify the positive health impact of community-level
programs.

REFERENCES

Acevedo-Garcia, D. (2001). Zip code-level risk factors for tuberculosis: Neighbor-
hood environment and residential segregation in New Jersey, 1985–1992.
American Journal of Public Health, 91, 734–741.
Azjen, I., & Fishbein, M. (1980). *Understanding attitudes and predicting social
behavior.* Englewood Cliffs, NJ: Prentice-Hall.
Bandura, A. (1977). Self-efficacy: Toward a unifying theory of behavioral change.
Psychological Review, 84(2), 191–215.
Bandura, A. (1997). *Self-efficacy: The exercise of control.* New York: Freeman.
Blumenthal, D. S., Sung, J., Williams, J., Liff, J., & Coates, R. (1995). Recruitment
and retention of subjects for a longitudinal cancer prevention study in an inner-
city Black community. *Health Services Research, 30*, 197–205.
Breslow, L. (1999). From disease prevention to health promotion. *Journal of the
American Medical Association, 281*, 1030–1033.
Carleton, R. A., Lasater, T. M., Assaf, A. R., Feldman, H. A., & McKinlay, S. (1995).
The Pawtucket Heart Health Program: Community changes in cardiovascular
risk factors and projected disease risk. *American Journal of Public Health,
85*, 777–785.

Cassel, J. (1964). Social science theory as a source of hypotheses in epidemiological research. *American Journal of Public Health, 54,* 1482–1488.

Centers for Disease Control and Prevention. (1999a). Compendium of HIV prevention interventions with evidence of effectiveness. Atlanta, GA: Department of Health and Human Resources.

Centers for Disease Control and Prevention. (1999b). CDC AIDS Community Demonstration Projects Research Group. Community-level HIV intervention in 5 cities: Final outcome data from the CDC AIDS Community Demonstration Projects. *American Journal of Public Health, 89,* 336–345.

Cohen, D. A., Scribner, R. A., & Farley, T. A. (2000). A structural model of health behavior: A pragmatic approach to explain and influence health behaviors at the population level. *Preventive Medicine, 30*(2), 146–154.

Cohen, D., Spear, S., Scribner, R., Kissinger, P., Mason, K., & Wildgen, J. (2000). "Broken windows" and the risk of gonorrhea. *American Journal of Public Health, 90,* 230–236.

COMMIT Research Group. (1995a). Community Intervention Trial for Smoking Cessation (COMMIT): I. Cohort results from a four-year community intervention. *American Journal of Public Health, 85,* 183–192.

COMMIT Research Group. (1995b). Community Intervention Trial for Smoking Cessation (COMMIT): II. Changes in adult cigarette smoking prevalence. *American Journal of Public Health, 85,* 193–200.

Crosby, R. A., DiClemente, R. J., Wingood, G. M., Harrington, K., Davies, S. L., Hook, E. W., et al. (2002). African American adolescent females' membership in community organizations is associated with STD/HIV-protective behaviors: A prospective analysis. *Journal of Epidemiological Community Health.*

Crosby, R. A., DiClemente, R. J., Wingood, G. M., Harrington, K., Davies, S. L., & Malow, R. (2002). African American adolescent females' membership in social organizations is associated with protective behavior against HIV infection. *Ethnicity and Disease, 12,* 186–189.

DiClemente, C. C., & Prochaska, J. O. (1998). Toward a comprehensive, transtheoretical model of change: Stages of change and addictive behaviors. In W. R. Miller & N. Heather (Eds.), *Treating addictive behaviors applied clinical psychology* (2nd ed., pp. 3–24). New York: Plenum Press.

Diez-Roux, A. V., Nieto, F. J., Muntaner, C., Tyroler, H. A., Comstock, G. W., Shahar, E., et al. (1997). Neighborhood environments and coronary heart disease: A multilevel analysis. *American Journal of Epidemiology, 146*(1), 48–63.

Emmons, K. M. (2000). Health behaviors in a social context. In L. F. Berkman & I. Kawachi (Eds.), *Social epidemiology* (pp. 242–266). New York: Oxford University Press.

Farquhar, J. W. (1978). The community-based model of life style intervention trials. *American Journal of Epidemiology, 108*(2), 103–111.

Fishbein, M. (1996). Editorial: Great expectations, or do we ask too much from community-level interventions? *American Journal of Public Health, 86,* 1075–1076.

Fortmann, S. P., Flora, J. A., Winkleby, M. A., Schooler, C., Taylor, C. B., & Farquhar, J. W. (1995). Community intervention trials: Reflections on the Stanford Five-City Project. *American Journal of Epidemiology, 142,* 576–586.

Friedman, S. R., Perlis, T., & Des Jarlais, D. C. (2001). Laws prohibiting over-the-counter syringe sales to injection drug users: Relations to population density, HIV prevalence, and HIV incidence. *American Journal of Public Health, 91,* 791–793.

Garrett, L. (1994). *The coming plague: Newly emerging diseases in a world out of balance.* New York: Farrar, Straus & Giroux.

Green, S. B. (1997). The advantages of community-randomized trials for evaluating lifestyle modification. *Controlled Clinical Trials, 18,* 506–513.

Green, S. B., Corle, D. K., Gail, M. H., Mark, S. D., Pee, D., Freedman, L. S., et al. (1995). Interplay between design and analysis for behavioral intervention trials with community as the unit of randomization. *American Journal of Epidemiology, 142,* 587–593.

Hennekens, C. H., & Buring, J. E. (1987). *Epidemiology in medicine.* Boston: Little, Brown.

Holtgrave, D. R., Crosby, R. A., DiClemente, R. J., Wingood, G. M., & Gayle, J. A. (2002). Social capital as a predictor AIDS cases, STD rates and adolescent sexual risk behavior prevalence: A state-level analysis, U.S.A., 1999. Presented at the XIV International AIDS Conference, Barcelona, Spain. Abstract published in conference proceedings (abstract no. THOrD1493).

Kaplan, G. A., Pamuk, E. R., Lynch, J. W., Cohen, R. D., & Balfour, J. L. (1996). Inequality in income and mortality in the United States: Analysis of mortality and potential pathways. *British Medical Journal, 312,* 999–1003.

Kawachi, I., Kennedy, B., & Glass, R. (1999). Social capital and self-rated health: A contextual analysis. *American Journal of Public Health, 89,* 1187–1193.

Kawachi, I., Kennedy, B., Lochner, K., & Prothrow-Stith, D. (1997). Social capital, income inequality, and mortality. *American Journal of Public Health, 87,* 1491–1498.

Kegeles, S. M., Hays, R. B., & Coates, T. J. (1996). The Mpowerment project: A community-level HIV prevention intervention for young gay men. *American Journal of Public Health, 86,* 1129–1136.

Kelly, J. A., Murphy, D. A., Sikkema, K. J., McAuliffe, T. L., Roffman, R. A., Solomon, L. J., et al. and the Community HIV Prevention Research Collaborative. (1997). Randomised, controlled, community-level HIV-prevention intervention for sexual-risk behaviour among homosexual men in US cities. *The Lancet, 350,* 1500–1504.

Kelly, J. A., St. Lawrence, J., Stevenson, Y., Hauth, A. C., Kalichman, S. C., Diaz, Y. E., et al. (1992). Community AIDS/HIV risk reduction: The effects of endorsements by popular people in three cities. *American Journal of Public Health, 82,* 1483–1489.

Koepsell, T. D., Diehr, P. H., Cheadle, A., & Kristal, A. (1995). Invited commentary: Symposium on community intervention trials. *American Journal of Epidemiology, 142,* 594–598.

Kreuter, M. W., & Lezin, N. A. (2002). Social capital theory: Implications for community-based health promotion. In R. J. DiClemente, R. A. Crosby, & M. C. Kegler (Eds.), *Emerging theories in health promotion practice and research* (pp. 228–254). San Francisco: Jossey-Bass/Wiley.

Lauby, J. L., Smith, P. J., Stark, M., Person, B., & Adams, J. (2000). A community-level HIV prevention intervention for inner-city women: Results of the Women and Infants Demonstration Projects. *American Journal of Public Health, 90,* 216–222.

Link, B. G., & Phelan, J. (1995). Social conditions as fundamental causes of disease [Special issue]. *Journal of Health and Social Behavior,* 80–94.

Luepker, R. V., Murray, D. M., Jacobs, D. R., Mittlemark, M. B., Bracht, N., Carlaw, R., et al. (1994). Community education for cardiovascular disease prevention: Risk factor changes in the Minnesota Heart Health Program. *American Journal of Public Health, 84,* 1383–1393.

Lynch, J. W., Kaplan, G. A., Pamuk, E. R., Cohen, R. D., Heck, K. E., Balfour, J. L., et al. (1998). Income inequality and mortality in metropolitan areas of the United States. *American Journal of Public Health, 88,* 1074–1080.

McKinlay, J. B. (1974). A case for refocusing upstream: The political economy of illness. In P. Conrad & R. Kern (Eds.), *The sociology of health and illness: Critical perspectives* (3rd ed., pp. 502–516). New York: St. Martin's Press.

McLeroy, K. R., Bibeau, D., Steckler, A., & Glanz, K. (1988). An ecological perspective on health promotion programs. *Health Education Quarterly, 15,* 351–377.

Murray, D. M. (1995). Design and analysis of community trials: Lessons from the Minnesota Heart Health Program. *American Journal of Epidemiology, 142,* 569–575.

Murray, D. M. (1998). *Design and analysis of group-randomized trials.* New York: Oxford University Press.

O'Campo, P., Xue, X., Wang, M., & Coughy, M. O. (1997). Neighborhood risk factors for low birth weight in Baltimore: A multilevel analysis. *American Journal of Public Health, 87,* 1113–1118.

Prochaska, J. O., DiClemente, C. C., Velicer, W. F., & Rossi, J. S. (1993). Standardized, individualized, interactive, and personalized self-help programs for smoking cessation. *Health Psychology, 12,* 399–405.

Putnam, R. D. (2000). *Bowling alone: The collapse and revival of American community.* New York: Touchstone.

Ramirez-Valles, J., Zimmerman, M. A., & Newcomb, M. D. (1998). Sexual risk behavior among youth: Modeling the influence of prosocial activities and socioeconomic factors. *Journal of Health and Social Behavior, 39,* 237–253.

Rietmeijer, C. A., Kane, M. S., Simons, P. Z., Corby, N. H., Wolitski, R. J., Higgins, D. L., et al. (1996). Increasing the use of bleach and condoms among injecting drug users in Denver: Outcomes of a targeted, community-level HIV prevention program. *AIDS, 10,* 291–298.

Robert, S. A. (1998). Community-level socioeconomic status effects on adult health. *Journal of Health and Social Behavior, 39*(1), 18–37.

Rogers, E. M. (1995). *Diffusion of innovations* (4th ed.). New York: Free Press.

Rose, G. (1985). Sick individuals and sick populations. *International Journal of Epidemiology, 14*(1), 32–38.

Rose, G. (1992). *The strategy of preventive medicine.* New York: Oxford University Press.

Runyan, D. K., Hunter, W. M., Socolar, R. R., Amaya-Jackson, L., English, D., Landsverk, J., et al. (1998). Children who prosper in unfavorable environments: The relationship to social capital. *Pediatrics, 101,* 12–18.

Schinke, S. P., Orlandi, M. A., & Cole, K. C. (1992). Boys and girls clubs in public housing developments: Prevention services for youth at risk. *Journal of Comparative Psychology, 28,* 118–128.

Sikkema, K. J., Kelly, J. A., Winett, R. A., Solomon, L. J., Cargill, V. A., Roffman, R. A., et al. (2000). Outcomes of a randomized community-level HIV prevention intervention for women living in 18 low-income housing developments. *American Journal of Public Health, 90,* 57–63.

Susser, M., & Susser, E. (1996). Choosing a future for epidemiology: Eras and paradigms. *American Journal of Public Health, 86,* 668–673.

Sweat, M. D., & Denison, J. A. (1995). Reducing HIV incidence in developing countries with structural and environmental interventions. *AIDS, 9*(Suppl. A), S251–S257.

Syme, S. L. (1996). Rethinking disease: Where do we go from here? *Annals of Epidemiology, 6,* 463–468.

Winkleby, M. A., Taylor, C. B., Jatulis, D., & Fortmann, S. P. (1996). The long-term effects of a cardiovascular disease prevention trial: The Stanford Five-City Project. *American Journal of Public Health, 86,* 1773–1779.

Chapter 10

CARDIOVASCULAR RISK-REDUCTION COMMUNITY INTERVENTION TRIALS

Sharon K. Davis

Beginning in the early 1970s, conventional wisdom guided by theoretical concepts and new scientific information ushered in a new wave of community-based randomized controlled trials designed to comprehensively lower multiple behavioral risk factors associated with the onset of cardiovascular disease; these included the Stanford Five-City Project (Farquhar, Fortmann, Maccoby, et al., 1985), the Minnesota Heart Health Program (Blackburn, Luepker, Kline, et al., 1984) and the Pawtucket Heart Health Program (Carleton, Lasater, Assaf, Lefebre, & McKinlay, 1987). These were investigator-initiated research and demonstration studies that included different aspects of health-promotion education as the primary intervention tool delivered through multiple channels. Various iterations have emerged over the past 35 years; however, the basic premise remains the same: Risk reduction intervention at the community-level will create a diffusion effect that will positively alter individual and subsequent community health by lowering the overall incidence of heart attacks and strokes.

The first generation of community-based intervention trials were large in scope and long term in duration, ranging from 10 to 14 years (Stone, 1991). Each adopted a clinical trial approach with community randomization assignments to treatment and control groups. The incongruent nature of this quasi-experimental design precluded the ability of investigators to create a truly "controlled" environment, which in large part contributed to unavoidable modest or negative results (Carleton, Lasater, Assaf, et al., 1995; Farquhar, Fortmann, Flora, et al., 1990; Luepker, Murray, Jacobs, et al., 1994). Despite less-than-anticipated outcomes, lessons learned from these initial intervention studies helped shape the development of subsequent, more successful second-generation projects with implications gleaned for a potentially new wave of targeted community intervention trials. The objective of this chapter is to provide insights regarding conceptual and methodological issues associated with community-based cardiovascular disease risk-reduction intervention trials by discussing (a) the historical context that contributed to the development and implementation of such studies in the United States, (b) key components of first-generation trials and adaptation of second-generation iterations, and (c) implications for future directions.

HISTORICAL BACKGROUND

All social change, including that related to public health, is rooted in, and influenced by, public policy decisions. So, too, was the case for a community-wide approach to the primary prevention of cardiovascular disease in the United States. The following discussion illustrates this point.

In 1900, as illustrated in chapter 1 at Table 1.1, the top three causes of death in the United States were infectious diseases (pneumonia and influenza, tuberculosis, diarrhea and enteritis) with disease of the heart following fourth. Fifty years later, diseases of the heart and stroke had shifted upward in rank to the first and third leading causes of death, respectively, and have continually maintained these positions. The National Heart, Lung, and Blood Institute (NHLBI) convened a task force in the late 1950s to ascertain the etiology associated with the epidemic shift in cardiovascular disease (White, Sprague, & Stamler, 1959). Evidence suggested an association with post–World War II increases in adverse health behaviors, including high-fat diets and smoking that lead to obesity, elevated blood cholesterol, and elevated blood pressure. Policy decisions were made to allocate funds to the development of an observational population-based epidemiologic study—the Framingham Heart Study—designed to determine the pathogenesis and prospects for early detection of cardiovascular disease. Evidence derived from this study established a scientific link between adverse lifestyle behaviors and the etiology of heart attacks and strokes (Feinleib, 1996).

Based on these findings, initial funds were allocated to the U.S. Veterans Administration, health care system during the 1960s to intervene on high-risk individuals using a medical model (Veterans Administration [VA], Cooperative Study Group, 1967). Research findings demonstrated the efficacy of intervening on single risk factors such as high blood pressure. A subsequent policy decision by the NHLBI Task Force recommended the initiation of intervention trials designed to comprehensively address multiple risk factors. The clinic-based Multiple Risk Factor Intervention Trial (MRFIT) was funded in 1972 and was based on a traditional individual-level medical model. Like the VA trials, it was focused on individuals and was not designed to address primary prevention or reduction of adverse lifestyle risk factors on a population-wide basis. Intervention results proved somewhat favorable but, not surprisingly, were less effective in terms of addressing excess cardiovascular risk at the community level (MRFIT Research Group, 1982).

Funded in 1970, the Stanford Three-Community Study was the first prototype in the United States designed to measure and demonstrate the effectiveness of a multiple cardiovascular-disease risk-reduction community-education intervention trial. Two years of research demonstrated significant net improvements in the reduction of plasma cholesterol levels, blood pressure levels, and smoking rates in intervention cities over control cities (Farquhar, Maccoby, Wood, et al., 1977). Positive findings from this study, coupled with results from the similarly designed North Karelia intervention trial in Finland (Puska, Tuomilehto, & Salonen, 1981), were the catalyst for the NHLBI Task Force to recommend broader, long-term U.S. research and demonstration projects designed to comprehensively field-test the effectiveness of educational interventions on multiple-risk-factor reduction at the community level (Stone, 1991). Three projects were subsequently funded in different regions of the country.

First-Generation Community-Based Intervention Trials

Funded in 1978, the Stanford Five-City Project evolved from the initial Three-City Community Project and included two intervention cities and two control cities. In a third city, investigators monitored changes in heart attack and stroke morbidity and mortality but did not conduct surveys as in the other two control cities. The cities were located in northern California (Farquhar et al., 1985). The Minnesota Heart Health Program, the largest of the three, was funded in 1980 and included three intervention cities and three control cities located in Minnesota and the Dakotas (Blackburn et al., 1984). The Pawtucket Heart Health Program, also funded in 1980, included one intervention city in Rhode Island and one control city in Massachusetts (Carleton et al., 1987).

CONCEPTUAL AND THEORETICAL DESIGN

The establishment of the link between cardiovascular disease and potentially preventable risk factors was the stimulus to field-test programs designed to demonstrate the ability of broad-based health education strategies to arrest negative health behaviors at the community level. Based on this unifying premise, all three studies addressed risk reduction through the prevention of cigarette smoking, elevated blood pressure, high-fat diet, obesity, and physical inactivity, using the dissemination of health education information as the intervention. The intervention was long term, lasting from 5 to 8 years, and included multiple channels of communication, from print and electronic media to interpersonal direct methods. Each project included a multidisciplinary research team of individuals with backgrounds in medicine, public health, communication, nutrition, exercise physiology, and psychology.

The design of these first-generation studies was based on an amalgam of theoretical social-learning paradigms, including community-health education, infused with community mobilization and activation, social marketing, and diffusion of innovation (Shea & Basch, 1990). It was assumed that personal health behavior was the overriding influence that contributed to the development of cardiovascular disease and that the combination of these elements, with health education as the core, would be an effective primary intervention tool with which to modify risk behaviors within communities. The overriding hypothesis was that exposure to risk-reduction education would result in risk modification at the individual level with a dose-response effect, thus ameliorating multiple risk factors at the community level and leading to a reduction of cardiovascular morbidity and mortality.

Each project included a research design that called for randomization of communities to treatment or control groups, matched on size and demographic composition and with nonoverlapping media boundaries. The general premise was that the concentration of preventive efforts on high-risk adults through the traditional medical model, such as MRFIT, would not capture youth and young adults who may exhibit risky behaviors that ultimately would contribute to excess risk at the community level (MRFIT Research Group, 1982). It was theorized that a broader public health approach would be more effective in that all ages and segments of the target community would be exposed to sustained intervention over a prolonged period of time. In addition, unlike the individual-based medical model, the primary aim of this broader population-based approach was to prevent or reduce adverse health behaviors that contributed to heart attack and stroke, rather than to treat the cardiovascular events after they occurred.

Formative evaluation—that is, evaluation conducted during the project in order to improve the project's methods—was an integral part of the overall evaluation. The evaluation of intervention effects was based on cross-sectional and cohort surveys among a random sample of individuals within a given household who ranged in age from 12 to 74 years. Surveys were conducted in both treatment and control communities in each of the projects with differing intervals for repeat measures. Changes in morbidity and mortality were also assessed through epidemiologic surveillance of fatal and nonfatal heart attacks and strokes in treatment and control communities. Annual budgets ranged from $1 million to $1.5 million throughout the duration of each project (Goodman, Wheeler, & Lee, 1995).

Methodological Issues

Despite the thoughtful nature of these well-conducted, rigorous trials, each produced modest or negative outcome results (Winkleby, 1994). Strong favorable secular increases in health knowledge and declines in smoking, blood pressure, and physical inactivity, for instance, were observed in the Stanford Project for both the treatment cities and the control cities, thus precluding the ability to detect statistically significant intervention effects (Farquhar et al., 1990). Results in the Minnesota and Pawtucket studies were similar in terms of the distribution of secular trends; findings were modest and within levels attributable to chance when comparing differences between treatment communities and control communities (Carleton et al., 1995; Luepker et al., 1994). Findings for the Pawtucket study are shown in Table 10.1 and are representative of the findings in each of these studies (the name of the comparison city in this study was not revealed because of a confidentiality agreement).

There were several plausible factors that may have contributed to the results observed in each of these community-based intervention trials. Two were perhaps the most overriding: competing secular trends and sample size associated with unit of analysis (Mittelmark, Hunt, Heath, & Schmid, 1993). These are discussed below.

Competing Secular Trends

Critical analyses of the study findings have been published by commentators and by the investigators (Feinlieb, 1996; Flora et al., 1995; Murray, 1995). It has been generally agreed that most of the targeted variables did in fact improve; however, the net magnitude of change was not statistically greater in the intervention communities when contrasted with the control communities. Unlike the pure scientific confines of a basic laboratory or clinical trial, community-based experimental research has the unique challenge of "blinding" entire control communities in order to test an intervention that perversely competes with a plethora of concurrent interventions offered by other, well-meaning public health programs. Such was the experience of the initial NHLBI community-intervention trials.

The "contaminating" health education messages that infiltrated control communities have been viewed as the chief cause of the weaker than anticipated findings of the intervention projects (Mittelmark et al., 1993). Indeed, the diffusion and acceleration of nationwide health promotion messages to the general population began as early as 1964, following the first Surgeon General's advisory report on smoking ("Smoking and Health," 1964). National and privately sponsored health campaigns and policy initiatives designed to alter adverse lifestyle health behaviors steadily increased during the 1970s and 1980s and continued throughout the 1990s—starting with antismoking policies (i.e., domestic airplane flights, cigarette warning labels, banned television advertisements), followed by NHLBI's National High Blood Pressure Education Program and the National Cholesterol Education Program, to name a few (Lenfant, 1986; Lieberman Research, 1991; NHLBI, 1973).

Beginning in the 1960s there were overall secular improvements in levels of risk factor awareness coinciding with antismoking initiatives,

TABLE 10.1 Characteristics of Respondents to Each of Six Cross-Sectional Surveys of Citizens Aged 18 through 64 Years in Pawtucket and the Comparison City

	City	Survey (Dates)					
		1 (1981–1982)	2 (1983–1984)	3 (1985–1986)	4 (1987–1989)	5 (1990–1991)	6 (1992–1993)
Respondents, no.	Paw-tucket	1,163	1,360	1,479	1,460	1,015	1,052
	Compar-ison	1,279	1,439	1,476	1,493	1,022	1,023
Response rate %	Paw-tucket	70	67	68	68	65	68
	Compar-ison	70	68	68	67	64	70
Age y, mean (*SD*)	Paw-tucket	39.1 (13.9)	39.3 (14.0)	38.9 (13.9)	39.1 (13.4)	38.5 (13.4)	38.7 (12.4)
	Compar-ison	40.1 (14.2)	39.4 (13.7)	39.0 (13.4)	38.9 (13.7)	39.3 (13.6)	39.6 (13.0)
Education ≥ 12 y, No. (%)	Paw-tucket	743 (64.8)	888 (65.3)	994 (67.2)	1,029 (70.6)	738 (72.9)	744 (70.7)
	Compar-ison	633 (49.8)	777 (54.0)	808 (54.8)	907 (60.8)	620 (60.8)	580 (56.7)
Median yearly household income, $	Paw-tucket	17,500	22,500	22,500	27,500	27,500	27,500
	Compar-ison	17,500	17,500	22,500	22,500	27,500	27,500
Resided ≥ 4 y in city, no. (%)	Paw-tucket	992 (85.5)	1,149 (84.5)	1,207 (81.6)	1,188 (81.4)	827 (81.5)	843 (80.1)
	Compar-ison	1,15 (90.3)	1,337 (92.9)	1,358 (92.0)	1,377 (92.2)	932 (91.2)	956 (93.5)
U.S. born, no. (%)	Paw-tucket	961 (82.6)	1,104 (81.2)	1,200 (81.1)	1,151 (78.8)	795 (78.3)	796 (75.7)
	Compar-ison	883 (69.1)	1,002 (69.6)	1,013 (68.6)	1,022 (68.5)	680 (66.5)	671 (65.6)
Female, no. (%)	Paw-tucket	651 (56.0)	795 (58.5)	860 (58.1)	794 (54.5)	570 (56.2)	614 (58.4)
	Compar-ison	762 (59.6)	854 (59.3)	875 (59.3)	861 (57.7)	560 (54.8)	598 (58.5)

Note: From Carleton, Lasater, Assaf, et al., 1995

with concomitant decreases in risk factor prevalence (Figure 10.1), including those targeted in the three NHLBI intervention projects (NHLBI, 1995). These observations support the idea that broad-based health promotion campaigns may have unintentionally altered the anticipated outcomes of the Stanford, Minnesota, and Pawtucket community intervention trials as evidenced by similar variable improvements in both treatment and control communities.

Unit-of-Analysis

Relative sample size was another important methodological factor, attributable to weak study findings stemming principally from the number of analytic units required to detect levels of statistical power. Unlike controlled clinical trials, where an individual is randomly assigned, the units of analysis in the three NHLBI studies were heterogeneous communities, with units of comparison ranging from $N = 1$ to $N = 3$. The average risk factor difference between treatment and control units at the end of the studies was approximately 2%–5%. The power of the design was consequently not sufficient to demonstrate statistical significance. Larger units of analysis were initially deemed necessary

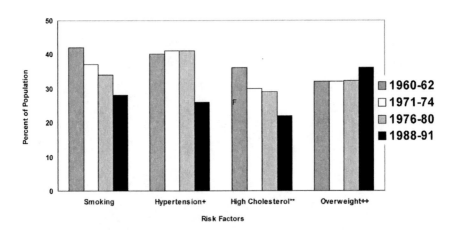

FIGURE 10.1 Trends in prevalence of risk factors, United States, 1960–1992.

Note: National Heart, Lung, and Blood Institute. Fact Book Fiscal Year 1994, National Institutes of Health, 1995

by investigators; however, budgetary constraints precluded the inclusion of additional communities.

The larger-scale 22-city, 4-year Community Intervention Trial for Smoking Cessation (COMMIT) was designed in part to address this problem (COMMIT, 1995a, 1995b). Eleven communities were randomly assigned to smoking intervention and 11 communities were assigned as controls. However, the results from this study were similarly modest and failed to achieve expected outcomes, owing to secular issues that eroded intervention effects as in the predecessor studies.

LESSONS LEARNED FOR FUTURE MODEL DEVELOPMENT

Despite the outcomes, much has been learned from the first wave of community-based intervention trials. The studies demonstrated the feasibility of implementing and conducting empirical health education research at the community level. Moreover, these intervention trials may have also contributed to the development of health-related policy initiatives and other population-based programs that resulted in overall improvements in the prevalence of risk factors in the general population.

Despite overall improvement in the last 40 years, not all segments of society have benefited equally. Subgroups of the population—particularly minorities and those who are poor—continue to experience disproportionately high rates of risk factors, morbidity, and mortality. Secular trends in levels of knowledge about risk factors associated with cardiovascular disease have not corrected this disparity. This pattern has been observed in the general U.S. population as well as in the treatment and control communities of the NHLBI studies. A pooled analysis of secular changes from 1980 through 1990 in acquired risk-factor knowledge, perceived risk-reduction knowledge, and interest in risk modification was conducted among respondents residing in treatment and control communities in the Stanford Five-City Project that participated in cross-sectional surveys in 1980, 1985, and 1990 (Davis, Winkleby, & Farquhar, 1995). There were significant overall increases in levels of knowledge, with a high level of interest in risk modification maintained over the decade (Figure 10.2). However, individuals with lower educational attainment experienced low to no improvements in levels of knowledge compared to improvements among those with more years of education (Figure 10.3). Despite this trend, the level of interest in risk modification remained equally high among

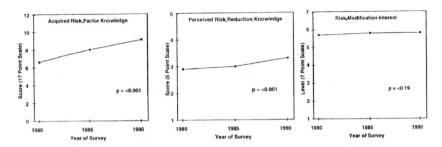

FIGURE 10.2   Overall trends over time in acquired cardiovascular disease risk factor knowledge, perceived risk reduction knowledge, and risk modification interest, Stanford Five-City Project, 1980–1990.

Note: Reprinted from the *American Journal of Preventive Medicine,* Volume II, by S. K. Davis, M. A. Winkleby, & J. W. Farquhar, Increasing disparity in knowledge of cardiovascular disease risk factors and risk reduction strategies by socioeconomic status: Implications for policymakers, pp. 318–323. Copyright, 1995. With permission from the *American Journal of Preventive Medicine* Inc.

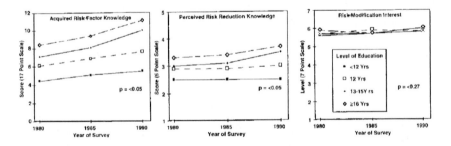

FIGURE 10.3   Trends over time by level of education in acquired cardiovascular disease risk factor knowledge, perceived risk reduction knowledge, and risk modification interest, Stanford Five-City Project, 1980–1990.

Note: Reprinted from the *American Journal of Preventive Medicine,* Volume II, by S. K. Davis, M. A. Winkleby, & J. W. Farquhar, Increasing disparity in knowledge of cardiovascular disease risk factors and risk reduction strategies by socioeconomic status: Implications for policymakers, pp. 318–323. Copyright, 1995. With permission from the *American Journal of Preventive Medicine* Inc.

respondents, regardless of the level of education. This suggests that health education may not have been effective in penetrating all segments of the community.

A similar pattern is also present in terms of secular trends in the distribution and prevalence of cardiovascular disease risk factors. Figure 10.1 depicts overall declines in the prevalence of cigarette smoking in the general U.S. population (NHLBI, 1995). Although improvement has occurred over time, the prevalence of cigarette-smoking African American men remains higher than in White men (NHLBI, 2000). Hypertension also remains significantly higher in African American men and women when compared to other racial and ethnic groups (NHLBI, 2000). Heart attack and stroke incidence and mortality parallel these observations (NHLBI, 2000).

In summary, subsequent community-based intervention trials should be modeled on lessons learned from first-generation studies but scaled down and targeted to discrete population subgroups within community neighborhoods that exhibit higher prevalence rates of modifiable risk factors.

SECOND-GENERATION COMMUNITY-BASED INTERVENTION TRIALS

Unlike their predecessors, smaller second-generation community trials on heart attack and stroke prevention report positive outcomes. Moreover, net effects are being achieved with a reduced budget and shorter duration to intervention exposure. The investigator-initiated Bootheel Heart Health Project provides such an example. This project was implemented in 6 counties in Missouri and used exercise groups, heart-healthy cooking demonstrations, and several risk-reduction education components as interventions (Brownson et al., 1996). Study subjects were exposed to interventions over a 3-year period. The investigators intentionally selected this particular area of Missouri as the location for the intervention because of the demographic characteristics of the region. The area is rural and has a high concentration of African American residents who are medically underserved and have high rates of poverty and low levels of educational attainment. The investigators reported significant population-wide improvement in fruit and vegetable consumption and prevalence of cholesterol screening. Improvements in physical activity, smoking, fruit and vegetable consumption, weight, and cholesterol screening were also reported in African Americans.

Unlike the previous studies, Bootheel incorporated coalition-building that guided the development of tailored community interventions within counties. Individual behavior change was evaluated as the primary unit of analysis rather than the community. The presence of a health coalition in a community was also used as an indicator to determine the degree of intervention exposure as opposed to random assignments of individuals or communities to treatment and control groups. Counties with a low coalition presence were compared to those with a higher degree of coalition-building to evaluate the effect of interventions on risk-factor behavior change. Positive changes resulted from the project at a relatively low annual cost of approximately $105,000. Evaluation expenses were minimized by collecting self-reported behavioral estimates and by limiting physiologic indicators.

The South Carolina Heart to Heart Project is an example of another second-generation cardiovascular community-based risk reduction program that has demonstrated success in yielding positive study outcomes (Croft et al., 1994). Although not focused on cardiovascular risk-reduction, another recently successful community-wide project aimed at HIV risk-factor behavior change further supports the concept that adapting intervention projects to the existing milieu of a community reduces the logistical and methodological complexities inherent in community-based research and demonstration projects (CDC, 1999).

SUMMARY AND IMPLICATIONS FOR FUTURE DIRECTIONS

Lessons learned from the first generation of cardiovascular risk-reduction community-based projects provide valuable insights with which to guide investigators in the development of subsequent iterations. Indeed, the community is not a laboratory or clinical trial venue in which subjects are blinded or randomly assigned to treatment and control groups. Rather, a given community is fluid and heterogeneous and includes individuals (not "subjects") with varying levels of receptivity to intervention exposure and varying dose-response risk reduction effects. The first wave of community trials, in conjunction with public health policy initiatives, has resulted in overall improvements in the overall levels of smoking, elevated cholesterol, elevated blood pressure, and physical activity. Excess risks, nevertheless, continue to exist in specific population subgroups. Second-generation projects are incorporating methodology concepts that allow flexible input and goal-setting by utilizing community conduits such as coalitions. More formative research is needed to elucidate the aggregate social and individual constraints that contribute to the prevalence of risky adverse health behaviors. Third-generation intervention trials should adopt contemporary models and move toward understanding potential pathways associated with risk factor prevalence that incorporate interventions designed to ameliorate such causal factors.

REFERENCES

Blackburn, H., Luepker, R. V., Kline, F. G., Bracht, N., Carlaw, R., Jacobs, D., et al. (1984). The Minnesota Heart Health Program: A research and demonstration project in cardiovascular disease prevention. In J. D. Matarazzo, S. M. Weiss, J. A. Herd, N. E. Miler, & S. M. Weiss (Eds.), *Behavioral health: A handbook of health enhancement and disease prevention.* New York: Wiley.

Brownson, R. C., Smith, C. A., Pratt, M., Mack, N. E., Jackson-Thompson, J., Dean, C. G., et al. (1996). Preventing cardiovascular disease through community-based risk reduction: The Bootheel Heart Health Project. *American Journal of Public Health, 86,* 206–213.

Carleton, R. A., Lasater, T. M., Assaf, A. R., Feldman, H. A., & McKinlay, S. (1995). The Pawtucket Heart Health Program: Community changes in cardiovascular risk factors and projected disease risk. *American Journal of Public Health, 85,* 777–785.

Carleton, R. A., Lasater, T. M., Assaf, A. R., Lefebre, R. C., & McKinlay, S. M. (1987). The Pawtucket Heart Health Program: An experiment in population-based disease prevention. *Rhode Island Medical Journal, 70,* 533–538.

CDC AIDS Community Demonstration Projects Research Group. (1999). *American Journal of Public Health, 89,* 336–345.

COMMIT Research Group Community Intervention Trial for Smoking Cessation I. (1995a). Cohort results from a four-year community intervention. *American Journal of Public Health, 85,* 183–192.

COMMIT Research Group Community Intervention Trial for Smoking Cessation II. (1995b). Changes in adult cigarette smoking prevalence. *American Journal of Public Health, 85,* 193–200.

Croft, J. B., Temple, S. P., Lankenau, B., Heath, G. W., Macera, C. A., Eaker, E. D., et al. (1994). Community intervention and trends in dietary fat consumption among Black and White adults. *Journal of the American Diet Association, 94,* 1284–1290.

Davis, S. K., Winkleby, M. A., & Farquhar, J. W. (1995). Increasing disparity in knowledge of cardiovascular disease risk factors and risk reduction strategies by socioeconomic status: Implications for policymakers. *American Journal of Preventive Medicine, 11,* 318–323.

Farquhar, J. W., Fortmann, S. P., Flora, J. A., Taylor, C. B., Haskell, W. L., Williams, P. T., et al. (1990). Effect of communitywide education on cardiovascular risk factors: The Stanford Five-City Project. *Journal of the American Medical Association, 264,* 359–365.

Farquhar, J. A., Fortmann, S. P., Maccoby, N., Haskell, W. L., Williams, P. T., Flora, J. A., et al. (1985). The Stanford Five-City Project: Design and methods. *American Journal of Epidemiology, 122,* 323–334.

Farquhar, J. W., Maccoby, N., Wood, P. D., Alexander, J. K., Breitrose, H., Brown, B. W., Jr., et al. (1977). Community education for cardiovascular health. *Lancet, 1,* 1192–1195.

Feinleib, M. (1996). Editorial: New directions for community intervention studies. *American Journal of Public Health, 86,* 1696–1997.

Fortmann, S. P., Flora, J. A., Winkleby, M. A., Schooler, C., Schooler, C., Taylor, C. B., et al. (1995). Community intervention trials: Reflections on the Stanford Five-City Project experience. *American Journal of Epidemiology, 142,* 576–586.

Goodman, R. M., Wheeler, F. C., & Lee, P. R. (1995). Evaluation of the Heart to Heart Project: Lessons learned from a community-based chronic disease prevention project. *American Journal of Health Promotion, 9,* 443–455.

Lenfant, C. A. (1986). A new challenge for America: The National Cholesterol Education Program. *Circulation, 73,* 855–856.

Lieberman Research. (1991). *A study of the impact of the 1991 Great American Smokeout: Summary. Gallup Organization.* New York: American Cancer Society.

Luepker, R. V., Murray, D. M., Jacobs, D. R., Bracht, N., Carlaw, R., Crow, R., et al. (1994). Community education for cardiovascular disease prevention: Risk factor changes in the Minnesota Heart Health Program. *American Journal of Public Health, 84,* 1383–1393.

Mittelmark, M. B., Hunt, M. K., Heath, G. W., & Schmid, T. L. (1993). Realistic outcomes: Lessons from community-based research and demonstration programs for the prevention of cardiovascular disease. *Journal of Public Health Policy, 14,* 455–462.

Multiple Risk Factor Intervention Trial Research Group. (1982). Multiple Risk Factor Intervention Trial: Risk factor changes and mortality results *Journal of the American Medical Association, 248,* 1465–1476.

Murray, D. A. (1995). Design and analysis of community trials: Lessons from the Minnesota Heart Health Program. *American Journal of Epidemiology, 142,* 569–575.

National Heart, Lung, and Blood Institute. (1973). Proceedings from the National Conference on High Blood Pressure Education. *DHEW Publication No. NIH in21386.* Washington, DC: DHEW.

National Heart, Lung, and Blood Institute. (1995, February). *Fact Book Fiscal Year 1994.* Washington, DC: National Institutes of Health.

Puska, P., Tuomilehto, J., & Salonen, J. (1981). The North Karelia Project: Evaluation of a comprehensive programme for control of cardiovascular diseases in 1972–1977 in North Karelia. Copenhagen, Denmark: World Health Organization.

Shea, S., & Basch, C. E. (1990). A review of five major community-based cardiovascular prevention programs. Part I: Rationale, design, and theoretical framework. *American Journal of Health Promotion, 4,* 203–213.

Smoking and Health: Report of the Advisory Committee to the Surgeon General. (1964). Washington, DC: U.S. Department of Health, Education, and Welfare.

Stone, E. J. (1991). Comparison of NHLBI Community-based cardiovascular research studies. *Journal of Health Education, 22,* 134–136.

Veterans Administration Cooperative Study Group on Hypertensive Agents. (1967). Effect of treatment on morbidity in hypertension: Results in patients with diastolic blood pressure averaging 115 through 129 mmHG. *Journal of the American Medical Association, 202,* 1028–1034.

White, P. D., Sprague, H. B., & Stamler, J. (1959). *A statement on arteriosclerosis: Main cause of heart attacks and strokes.* New York: National Education Committee.

Winkleby, M. A. (1994). The future of community-based cardiovascular disease intervention studies. *American Journal of Public Health, 84,* 1369–1372.

Index

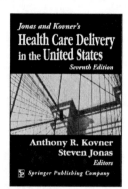

Springer Publishing Company

Linking Medical Care and Community Services

Practical Models for Bridging the Gap

Walter Leutz, PhD, Merwyn R. Greenlick, PhD, and Lucy Nonnenkamp, MA

How can a medical care system structure itself best to serve the total needs of the frail and disabled members of its population? Kaiser Permanente set out to answer this question. Its extraordinary 32-site demonstration program investigated the issues linking two systems (medical and long-term care) to improve how helping professionals and organizations can cooperate to assist people in their struggles to cope with chronic illness and disability.

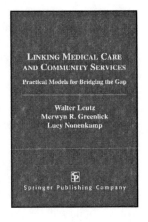

This book explores that potential collaboration between a wide range of service providers, such as doctors and hospitals, and community care agencies, including day care services, group homes, and family caregivers.

Contents:

2003   256pp   0-8261-1754-6   hard

536 Broadway, New York, NY 10012
Order Toll-Free: 877-687-7476 • Order On-line: www.springerpub.com